Evolving Crisis Standards of Care and Ongoing Lessons from COVID-19

Megan Snair, Aurelia Attal-Juncqua, and Scott Wollek, Rapporteurs

Forum on Medical and Public Health Preparedness for Disasters and Emergencies

Board on Health Sciences Policy

Health and Medicine Division

Proceedings of a Workshop Series

THE NATIONAL ACADEMIES PRESS   500 Fifth Street, NW   Washington, DC 20001

This activity was supported by contracts between the National Academy of Sciences and the Administration for Children and Families (contract no. HHS P233201400020B/75P00120F37103), the Assistant Secretary for Preparedness and Response (contract no. 75A50121P00089), the Centers for Disease Control and Prevention (contract no. 200-2011-38807/75D30120F00093), the Department of Homeland Security (contract no. HSHQDC-17-A-B0001/70RHAD18FR0000003), the Food and Drug Administration (contract no. 75F40120P00067), the National Highway Traffic Safety Administration (contract no. 693JJ921P000049), and the National Institutes of Health (contract no. HHSN263201800029I/HHSN26300026). Any opinions, findings, conclusions, or recommendations expressed in this publication do not necessarily reflect the views of any organization or agency that provided support for the project.

International Standard Book Number-13: 978-0-309-68879-6
International Standard Book Number-10: 0-309-68879-5
Digital Object Identifier: https://doi.org/10.17226/26573

Additional copies of this publication are available from the National Academies Press, 500 Fifth Street, NW, Keck 360, Washington, DC 20001; (800) 624-6242 or (202) 334-3313; http://www.nap.edu.

Copyright 2022 by the National Academy of Sciences. All rights reserved.

Printed in the United States of America

Suggested citation: National Academies of Sciences, Engineering, and Medicine. 2022. *Evolving crisis standards of care and ongoing lessons from COVID-19: Proceedings of a workshop series*. Washington, DC: The National Academies Press. https://doi.org/10.17226/26573.

The **National Academy of Sciences** was established in 1863 by an Act of Congress, signed by President Lincoln, as a private, nongovernmental institution to advise the nation on issues related to science and technology. Members are elected by their peers for outstanding contributions to research. Dr. Marcia McNutt is president.

The **National Academy of Engineering** was established in 1964 under the charter of the National Academy of Sciences to bring the practices of engineering to advising the nation. Members are elected by their peers for extraordinary contributions to engineering. Dr. John L. Anderson is president.

The **National Academy of Medicine** (formerly the Institute of Medicine) was established in 1970 under the charter of the National Academy of Sciences to advise the nation on medical and health issues. Members are elected by their peers for distinguished contributions to medicine and health. Dr. Victor J. Dzau is president.

The three Academies work together as the **National Academies of Sciences, Engineering, and Medicine** to provide independent, objective analysis and advice to the nation and conduct other activities to solve complex problems and inform public policy decisions. The National Academies also encourage education and research, recognize outstanding contributions to knowledge, and increase public understanding in matters of science, engineering, and medicine.

Learn more about the National Academies of Sciences, Engineering, and Medicine at **www.nationalacademies.org**.

Consensus Study Reports published by the National Academies of Sciences, Engineering, and Medicine document the evidence-based consensus on the study's statement of task by an authoring committee of experts. Reports typically include findings, conclusions, and recommendations based on information gathered by the committee and the committee's deliberations. Each report has been subjected to a rigorous and independent peer-review process and it represents the position of the National Academies on the statement of task.

Proceedings published by the National Academies of Sciences, Engineering, and Medicine chronicle the presentations and discussions at a workshop, symposium, or other event convened by the National Academies. The statements and opinions contained in proceedings are those of the participants and are not endorsed by other participants, the planning committee, or the National Academies.

Rapid Expert Consultations published by the National Academies of Sciences, Engineering, and Medicine are authored by subject-matter experts on narrowly focused topics that can be supported by a body of evidence. The discussions contained in rapid expert consultations are considered those of the authors and do not contain policy recommendations. Rapid expert consultations are reviewed by the institution before release.

For information about other products and activities of the National Academies, please visit www.nationalacademies.org/about/whatwedo.

PLANNING COMMITTEE ON EVOLVING CRISIS STANDARDS OF CARE AND LESSONS LEARNED[1]

ERIC TONER (*Chair*), Senior Scholar, Johns Hopkins University
ASHA DEVEREAUX, Senior Medical Officer, Sharp Coronado Hospital
MEGAN JEHN, Associate Professor, Arizona State University
ANUJ MEHTA, Pulmonary and critical care physician, Denver Health and Hospital Authority
GREGG S. MEYER, President, Community Division, and Executive Vice President, Value-Based Care, Mass General Brigham
MONICA E. PEEK, Associate Professor of Medicine, University of Chicago
JENNIFER PIATT, Deputy Director, Network for Public Health Law–Western Region Office
ERIN SERINO, Deputy Chief of Staff, Boston Emergency Medical Services
TENER GOODWIN VEENEMA, Contributing Scholar, Professor of Nursing, Johns Hopkins Center for Health Security, Johns Hopkins Bloomberg School of Public Health
MICHAEL WARGO, Vice President and Chief, Enterprise Preparedness and Emergency Operations, HCA Healthcare
SHANDIIN WOOD, Health Systems Epidemiologist and Tribal Liaison, New Mexico Department of Health
MATTHEW WYNIA, Director, University of Colorado Center for Bioethics and Humanities

Health and Medicine Division Staff

SCOTT WOLLEK, Forum Director
LISA BROWN, Senior Program Officer
AURELIA ATTAL-JUNCQUA, Program Officer
MICHAEL BERRIOS, Research Associate
KIMBERLY SUTTON, Senior Program Assistant
ANDREW M. POPE, Director, Board on Health Sciences Policy

---

[1] The National Academies of Sciences, Engineering, and Medicine's planning committees are solely responsible for organizing the workshop, identifying topics, and choosing speakers. The responsibility for the published Proceedings of a Workshop rests with the workshop rapporteurs and the institution.

Consultants

LAURA RUNNELS, LAR Consulting
KELLY SCHENK, LAR Consulting
MEGAN SNAIR, SGNL Solutions
JUSTIN SNAIR, SGNL Solutions

Reviewers

This Proceedings of a Workshop Series was reviewed in draft form by individuals chosen for their diverse perspectives and technical expertise. The purpose of this independent review is to provide candid and critical comments that will assist the National Academies of Sciences, Engineering, and Medicine in making each published proceedings as sound as possible and to ensure that it meets the institutional standards for quality, objectivity, evidence, and responsiveness to the charge. The review comments and draft manuscript remain confidential to protect the integrity of the process.

We thank the following individuals for their review of this proceedings:

JAMES G. HODGE, Peter Kiewit Foundation Professor of Law, Director of the Center for Public Health Law and Policy, Sandra Day O'Connor College of Law, Arizona State University
JEFFREY UPPERMAN, Professor and Chair, Department of Pediatric Surgery, Vanderbilt University
MATTHEW WATSON, Senior Analyst, Johns Hopkins Center for Health Security; Senior Research Associate Johns Hopkins Bloomberg School of Public Health

Although the reviewers listed above provided many constructive comments and suggestions, they were not asked to endorse the content of the proceedings nor did they see the final draft before its release. The review of this proceedings was overseen by **ROBERTA LAVIN**, FAAN Professor and Ph.D. Program Director at the University of New Mexico, College of Nursing. She was responsible for making certain that an independent examination of this proceedings was carried out in accordance with the standards of the National Academies and that all review comments were carefully considered. Responsibility for the final content rests entirely with the rapporteurs and the National Academies.

Contents

ABBREVIATIONS AND ACRONYMS   xi

1   INTRODUCTION   1
      Organization of the Workshop, 3
      Organization of the Proceedings, 4

2   REFLECTIONS, INFLECTIONS, AND THE FUTURE   5
      The First 10 Years of Crisis Standards of Care, 5
      Three Scenarios of Crisis Standards of Care, 8
      Looking Back at Firsthand Experiences and Lessons Learned, 11

3   CONSIDERATIONS FOR STAFFING, EFFECTS ON THE
      WORKFORCE, AND FUTURE TRENDS   19
      Effects of COVID-19 on the Workforce, 19
      Promising Staffing Strategies and Future Directions, 25
      Reflections on the Nursing Crisis and Future Directions, 31

4   CRISIS STANDARDS OF CARE: FROM PLANS TO REALITY   33
      Setting the Stage, 33
      Implementation Case Stories, 34
      Exploring Challenges in Crisis Standards of Care, 39
      Reflections, 45

5 **LEGAL, ETHICAL, AND EQUITY CONSIDERATIONS FOR CRISIS STANDARDS OF CARE** 47
Liability Protections: Issues Around Making Triage Decisions, 47
Equity and the Allocation of Scarce Resources, 50
Reflections, 53

6 **LOOKING FORWARD** 57
Keynote Presentations, 57
Reflections on Challenges and Opportunities, 59
Looking to the Future, 68

REFERENCES 73

APPENDIXES
A Workshop Agendas 77
B Speaker Biosketches 87

Abbreviations and Acronyms

ASPR Office of the Assistant Secretary for Preparedness and Response

CDPHE Colorado Department of Public Health and Environment
CSC crisis standards of care

EMS emergency medical services

HHS U.S. Department of Health and Human Services

ICU intensive care unit

MRC Medical Reserve Corps

OCR Office for Civil Rights

PPE personal protective equipment

SOFA sequential organ failure assessment
SVI Social Vulnerability Index

1

Introduction

Crisis standards of care (CSC) planning began at the national level in 2009 during the H1N1 pandemic. Efforts included the publication of an Institute of Medicine Letter Report underlining the importance of having more guidance for health care institutions and providers. The dramatic experiences during Hurricane Katrina in New Orleans in 2005 were followed by significant concerns about the resiliency of our health care system when the 2009/2010 H1N1 pandemic arose. It quickly became clear that leaving some of these critical life-or-death decisions to chance or to be made by those under stress at the bedside, without protections or guidance, was no longer an option. From that point, several more consensus reports emerged through the National Academies of Sciences, Engineering, and Medicine, as well as ad hoc workshops on community engagement and lessons learned after 10 years of conversations, and this type of specialized planning matured around the country. While the focus and intensity of CSC planning by government officials and public health and health care leaders has ebbed and flowed over the years, numerous points throughout the COVID-19 pandemic have demonstrated the necessity of this type of crisis planning. Given the rise in firsthand experiences with allocation of scarce resources and questions of balancing patients adequately across a region during extended emergencies, the Forum on Medical and Public Health

Preparedness for Disasters and Emergencies identified the need to pull some of these lessons together to inform current and future efforts (see Box 1-1).[1]

BOX 1-1
Workshop Series Statement of Task

A planning committee of the National Academies of Sciences, Engineering, and Medicine will organize and conduct a series of public workshops on the topic of crisis standards of care (CSC) during public health emergencies, including lessons learned from the COVID-19 pandemic.

The COVID-19 pandemic overwhelmed the U.S. medical care system and supporting supply chains for medications and materials, which led to the widespread consideration of crisis standards of care (CSC) planning and selected implementation of key elements of the CSC framework in communities across the nation. This workshop series will consist of five sessions beginning with an overarching, introductory session that will explore the reexamination of definitions and recommendations first outlined in IOM's 2009 *Guidance for Establishing Crisis Standards of Care for Use in Disaster Situations: A Letter Report*. Subsequent workshops will examine the systems framework articulated in IOM's 2012 report *Crisis Standards of Care: A Systems Framework for Catastrophic Disaster Response,* with a particular attention on:

- Planning and implementation considerations:
  - Examine the role of key stakeholders groups, such as state governments, state and local health departments, hospitals and health care systems, and other stakeholders at the federal, state, local, tribal, and territorial levels in the implementation and communication of CSC.
  - Explore the types of data required to inform CSC triggers, the sources of such data, and the plans for creating the needed infrastructure to allow for better situational awareness, including, for example, disease reporting, surveillance data, hospital transfer data sharing, and how to best use electronic health records for the development of more effective clinical processes and operations.

---

[1] The planning committee's role was limited to planning the workshop, and this Proceedings of a Workshop has been prepared by the workshop rapporteurs as a factual summary of what occurred at the workshop. Statements, recommendations, and opinions expressed are those of individual presenters and participants and are not necessarily endorsed or verified by the National Academies of Sciences, Engineering, and Medicine, and they should not be construed as reflecting any group consensus.

- Understand how jurisdictions may have changed their attitudes and beliefs about CSC planning as a result of COVID-19.
- Understand how the public's attitudes and beliefs about CSC have changed as a result of COVID-19.
• Legal, regulatory, and equity considerations:
- Explore concerns surrounding emergency declarations, invocation, duties to care, interjurisdictional challenges, discrimination, licensure and scope of practice, risks of liability, documentation, and mitigation.
- Discuss ethics, palliative care, mental health, and other crosscutting themes.
• Staffing considerations:
- Explore the challenges and strategic opportunities for operational considerations and staffing needs during the implementation of CSC.
- Define the roles and responsibilities of these stakeholders.
- Describe operational considerations associated with the development and implementation of CSC plans.
- Examine critical care triage teams, their role, protocols, and tools, specifically pertaining to prognostics systems.
- Provide brief descriptions of templates that outline the specific functions and tasks for each stakeholder when allocating scarce resources in response to a disaster.
- Review staff responsibilities adjustments, capabilities for just-in-time training, provision of hazard pay, adequate time off, childcare and other benefits for staff, and using health care coalitions to ensure appropriate transfer of patients between hospitals.

The series will conclude with a workshop discussing how to effectively take advantage of identified opportunities and how to best implement improvements in CSC.

ORGANIZATION OF THE WORKSHOP

This workshop series was organized and held virtually as five webinars throughout October and November 2021.[2] The first workshop introduced the concept of CSC and focused on reflections and opportunities for the future. The second workshop recounted ongoing lessons from the COVID-19 pandemic in terms of staffing and workforce needs. The third

---

[2] https://www.nationalacademies.org/our-work/evolving-crisis-standards-of-care-and-lessons-learned-a-workshop-series (accessed January 5, 2022).

workshop examined planning and the implementation of CSC plans at various levels. The fourth highlighted the legal, ethical, and equity considerations of CSC planning and what has been learned from the COVID-19 pandemic. The fifth and final workshop summarized discussion points across the previous meetings and offered key lessons in the different lanes of planning and highlighted opportunities for change.

ORGANIZATION OF THE PROCEEDINGS

This proceedings is organized into six chapters aligned with the individual webinars. Following this introductory chapter, Chapter 2 focuses on the initial CSC framework and looks back on its implementation in various scenarios. Chapter 3 highlights the staffing considerations and future trends that can inform planning and implementation. Chapter 4 covers CSC planning and implementation with examples from several jurisdictions. Chapter 5 reviews the lessons learned from COVID-19 with respect to legal, ethical, and equity considerations. As the final chapter, Chapter 6 brings together several key lessons and suggestions from various speakers to inform future planning and to identify areas with the greatest potential for positive change.

2

Reflections, Inflections, and the Future

The world has experienced numerous public health emergencies since 2012, when the first crisis standards of care (CSC) frameworks and concepts were released (IOM, 2012; Wilder-Smith and Osman, 2020). Reviewing the initial work and reports to gauge their merit and to determine where updates might be helpful is an important step forward when assessing this large body of work. This chapter reviews the framework and initial concepts developed around CSC, presents various scenarios where they might be used, and includes a description of the discussion that followed this workshop's presentation. These discussions highlight lessons learned from those working in the field over the last decade, in terms of what went well during implementation, as well as what is still needed to make future plans more resilient and to better support health care systems, clinicians, and other stakeholders during the next catastrophic emergency.

THE FIRST 10 YEARS OF CRISIS STANDARDS OF CARE

When the Forum on Medical and Public Health Preparedness for Disasters and Emergencies convened the workshop *Crisis Standards of Care: Ten Years of Successes and Challenges* in November 2019,[1] the first cases of COVID-19 were already appearing in Wuhan, China. Dan Hanfling, vice president of Technical Staff at In-Q-Tel, noted that this unfortunate pandemic experience has provided an opportunity to reexamine the CSC

---

[1] https://www.nap.edu/catalog/25767/crisis-standards-of-care-ten-years-of-successes-and-challenges (accessed January 5, 2022).

framework and its implementation as well as the successes and failures of current CSC approaches. Sharing a quote from a 2017 World Bank report, he said:

> Multiple pandemics, numerous outbreaks, thousands of lives lost and billions of dollars of national income wiped out—all since the turn of this century, in barely 17 years—and yet the world's investments in pandemic preparedness and response remain woefully inadequate. (World Bank Group, 2017)

To be clear, he added, "This finding was before COVID-19 arose."

Reviewing the last 10 years of work by the National Academies, Hanfling shared the original definition of CSC from the initial 2009 report: "A substantial change in usual health care operations and the level of care it is possible to deliver, which is made necessary by a pervasive (e.g., pandemic influenza) or catastrophic (e.g., earthquake, hurricane) disaster" (IOM, 2009). With the release of the 2012 and 2013 IOM reports came more focus on a systems framework and the identification of indicators and triggers. Hanfling commented on the mindset that CSC was more of a continuum, requiring movement from conventional care, to contingency surge, to crisis surge—not a switch to toggle on and off. He illustrated this through a graph representing a supply-and-demand curve for health care services (see Figure 2-1). By having enhanced preparedness and availability of resources, he said, the time available before entering the area under that

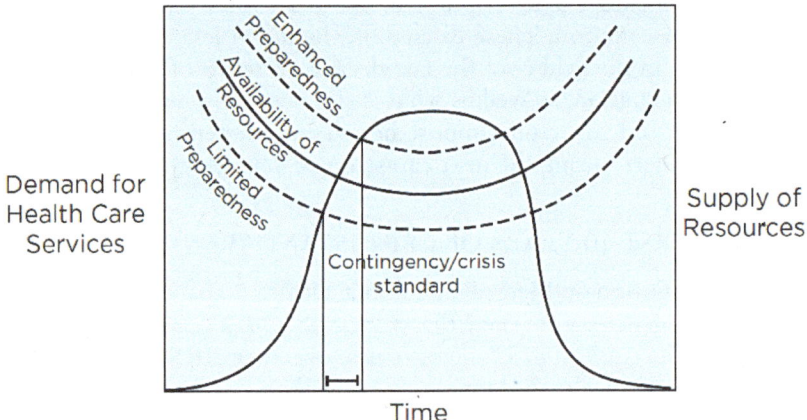

FIGURE 2-1 Demand for health care services and supply of resources as a function of time after disaster onset, taking into account care capacity as a function of time.
SOURCE: Dan Hanfling presentation, September 27, 2021. (Original source: IOM, 2012.)

curve is increased, and the area below the curve can be entered at a later point, allowing more time to operate under normal standards of care as the event progresses.

Taking the graphical representation a step further, Hanfling also shared a structural image resembling the Lincoln Memorial as a metaphor for the CSC framework (see Figure 2-2). He explained that the success of planning is built on engagement, education, ethical considerations, legal authorities, and information sharing, with all working together to improve performance. And while each of the pillars of hospital care, public health, emergency management, emergency medical services (EMS), and others are often operating within their own siloes, they all must coordinate to shift to standards of care that are still ethical and equitable across a city or region. He commented on the importance of being open to learning what works and making midcourse corrections when things are not working. For example, in the spring of 2020 in New York City, providers overrun by COVID-19 patients began to realize that early aggressive airway management and intubation was not as successful as initially thought. They instead shifted to other means of managing patients such as placing them prone to provide more oxygen.

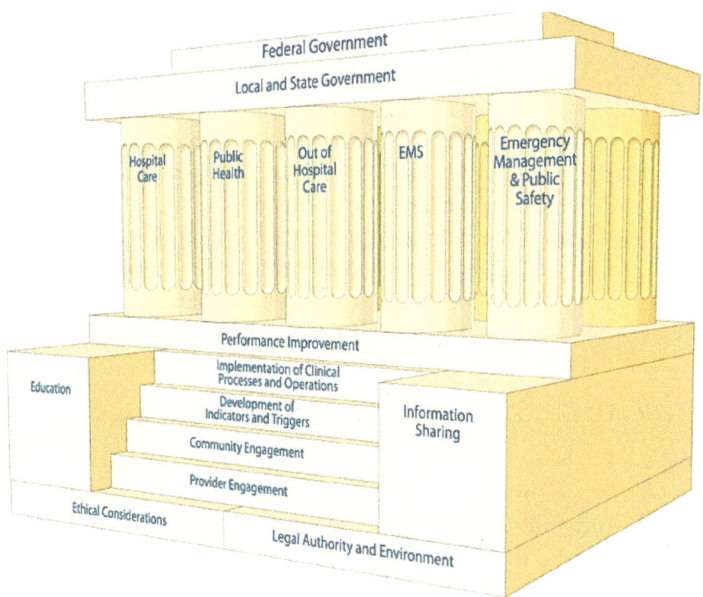

FIGURE 2-2 Structural metaphor resembling the Lincoln Memorial for CSC planning.
NOTE: EMS = emergency medical services.
SOURCE: Dan Hanfling presentation, September 27, 2021. (Original source: IOM, 2012.)

Hanfling reviewed where CSC stood in 2021, in terms of what worked for planning and what did not. He said the requirement for this type of catastrophic emergency planning has not been completely invalidated, the systems framework as designed is still relevant and can provide a solid foundation, and the nomenclature for terms and recommendations from the first 2009 report are still valid and necessary (IOM, 2009). He said this was important because more and more health care workers rightfully believe this will not be the last pandemic they will be a part of in their careers. However, he also had several examples of what did not work through this experience.

Hanfling said the multiple levels of dysfunctional government action that were seen across the country between February 2020 and September 2021 made it even more difficult for health care workers and planners to adequately respond. The clear inequities in disease burden and the effects of systemic racism also demonstrated a critical need to examine how the system can be changed to improve outcomes and equity. Finally, the lack of decision-support tools to assist in bedside clinical decision making was noticeable, especially in an ever-changing world of emerging data and new protocols for care.

Hanfling concluded that CSC planning is at an inflection point, and that the ethical framework, in the midst of a national crisis, demands some reconsideration in terms of accountability and reciprocity. Hanfling noted that while it is not clear if some of the available tools should actually be used at the point of care when resources are in high demand, what is clear is that the inherent inequities that have been illuminated throughout this crisis need to be given more attention and addressed at a systems level. This includes investment in capabilities, platforms, data analytics, and community engagement to provide as much situational awareness as possible so hospital systems and frontline care providers can make well-informed decisions about when the allocation of care delivery needs to be modified.

THREE SCENARIOS OF CRISIS STANDARDS OF CARE

Craig Vanderwagen, the first assistant secretary for preparedness and response (ASPR) within the U.S. Department of Health and Human Services (HHS), and founder and general manager of East West Protection, LLC, provided three different, successful scenarios to elucidate the range of situations that could call upon CSC planning.

Developing CSC Planning for Nationwide Hospitals

The first scenario refers to HCA Healthcare, a nationwide health system, and how it approached CSC in early March 2020 in response to

COVID-19. Vanderwagen reviewed HCA Heathcare's characteristics, noting it includes 200 hospitals nationwide and has a sophisticated planning and operational capability for preparedness. The issue of CSC had been lurking in the background for HCA Healthcare, but by February 2020 the leadership realized CSC challenges needed to be addressed in a systematic way. In March 2020, ASPR began working with HCA Healthcare and its lawyers, clinical staff, and chief medical officers to develop an effective CSC program that prioritized resource sparing[2] and contingency standards. He noted that the system preemptively developed a legal and ethical framework for crisis standards with transparency and accountability and operated in the context of legal stipulations.

Then, HCA Healthcare worked with medical staff to develop a triage system and set of processes. Systemwide, it was recognized that individual hospitals had their own governance committees and their own medical staff engaging with their communities and making decisions, so there was not an option for a one-size-fits-all approach, he explained. Instead, HCA Healthcare gave every hospital an operating set of guidelines that could be tailored to the reality of the communities and practices in which they operated. By the end of March 2020, every facility had embraced the notion of CSC, the governance boards approved it, and they all engaged with communities to discuss what it would mean for them. Medical and nursing staff had strong input into the processes that would be used, included triage and quality assurance.

Vanderwagen highlighted an interesting spinoff, as HCA Healthcare is supplied by an organization that supplies 1,600 hospitals nationwide. This organization also provides logistical support for the supply chains to most of those hospitals, Vanderwagen noted, so they also were involved in the CSC development process. That organization wanted to understand how it could support moving away from just-in-time supply chains and move toward a resource-sparing strategy. Over the last year and a half, he said, that organization has begun investing in manufacturing capacity for certain kinds of products that are known to be in short supply in this kind of event. Because of those investments, he said, this supply chain group can now be ahead of the preparedness curve and shorten the time spent under the curve, as previously portrayed in Figure 2-1. This is the kind of forward and innovative thinking that needs to be encouraged and incentivized within all hospital systems, he said. HCA Healthcare viewed CSC as critical to the community good. It was willing and able to invest in that process, but not every hospital system can do that. All systems should be incentivized

---

[2] The process of maximizing the utility of supplies and material through conservation, substitution, reuse, adaptation, and reallocation.

to ensure they can take those kinds of steps toward multidisciplinary CSC planning, he concluded.

Deploying an Alternate Care Site in a Major Metropolitan Area

The second scenario involved the deployment of an alternate care site in the Boston area involving 20–30 hospitals banding together to take action. Beginning in late March 2020, hospitals in that community began to realize they needed to develop a strong contingency plan that focused on resource sparing so they could continue to manage the patient flow confronting them. They decided to set up alternate care sites to decompress their hospitals and support intensive care capability, he explained, but they wanted to do it in a way that was ethical and accountable. Given the fact that COVID-19 was thus far significantly affecting neighborhoods of color and the large homeless population in Boston, there were questions about how to deliver appropriate supports for these types of populations.

Vanderwagen explained that the program of care in the alternate care facility was designed around rehabilitation, noting that when patients came out of the intensive care unit (ICU), the system needed to be prepared to provide the right rehabilitation services to get the patients back into their community with their care managed appropriately. With this in mind, the effort involved community health providers and local long-term care facilities, though many were shut down at the time or not in business owing to the restrictions and stay-at-home orders. The hospitals did have strong support from the mayor and governor in terms of ensuring the supply chain throughout the process, Vanderwagen noted, which was helpful in getting what they needed.

For 8 weeks from April to June 2020, the alternate care site was able to serve 800 patients, including 100 homeless people. The hospitals were able to effectively provide rehab services and link the patients back to their community once they were discharged from the alternate care site. The system used a community-wide approach, employed equity as a basic principle, and linked the design to what those patients needed when they recovered. The hospitals also coordinated and clarified discharge criteria, so there were clear standards for admission and discharge.

Community Efforts to Develop Alternate Care Sites

The third scenario involves the community's effort in El Paso, Texas, that used its unity to meet the needs of the population, even without political support at the state level. The state did not have a CSC plan, Vanderwagen explained, but the significant surging of patients in El Paso during the first wave of the pandemic resulted in all hospitals being confronted with the need to conduct very aggressive resource-sparing strategies. Among those strategies was the use of an alternate care site, but there were concerns about the need for a common message to patients and the community about what the facility would be. He explained that the state wanted to ensure the community understood the alternate care site was not to be a depository for COVID-19 patients, but that it would be built around principles of equity and rehabilitation services to get recovered patients back into their home environment in the best shape possible.

The community did have strong political leadership and support at the local level from the mayor and the county judge executive, who supported hospitals collectively taking advantage of alternate care sites with common messaging and discharge criteria. This made the facility into a critically important resource, he added. He concluded that the site became a very successful transitional service, where people understood they were being cared for and in the right shape when sent home.

These three scenarios demonstrate a few important lessons, Vanderwagen concluded. First, community-wide planning is critical. Additionally, clinical participation in determining the standards of care and how resource sparing will be employed, as well as education in how that can be used creatively, are critically important. Alternate care sites can be very effective in a resource-sparing strategy. He noted a failure in this process at the national level, though, saying that the Army Corps of Engineers went too far and built too many facilities during the pandemic, and many went unused. He explained that joint community planning that includes all stakeholders can lead to much more effective use of the facilities that are built. Finally, he suggested the Centers for Medicare and Medicaid Services (CMS) think about how to provide incentives through payment to support this kind of resource-sparing strategy for hospitals and health care organizations.

LOOKING BACK AT FIRSTHAND EXPERIENCES AND LESSONS LEARNED

To take a deeper look at what has been learned over the past 10 years, Eric Toner, senior scholar at the Center for Health Security, Johns Hopkins University, introduced a panel of experts with firsthand experience in CSC planning and implementation. They introduced topics that are also discussed in further depth throughout this workshop series, including ethics and equity, staffing considerations and clinical issues, and legal lessons and accountability.

Ethics and Equity

Monica Peek, professor of medicine at the University of Chicago, believes that CSC planning has reached a tipping point. Experts had worked to gather information from the community about what was important, she said, but that information had not yet been translated to implementation when COVID-19 first emerged. She also pointed out that many thought leaders have emphasized the engagement of politicians and health care leaders to get the right buy-in and support, but she emphasized that there is a lot of work that can be done right now. She shared the quote "Every system is perfectly designed to get the results it gets," hinting that the inequities that have emerged throughout the pandemic are not singular, isolated mistakes or gaps, but instead demonstrate a more pervasive issue within the system.

In this case, she continued, the systems are designed for inequity. Peek called for designing systems using an ethical framework so people who have historically had less can have more, so outcomes are equitable, not equal. She added that people take for granted that everyone has equal access to goods, resources, and opportunities in their everyday lives, but there has been enough evidence to show that this is not the case. Peek emphasized that unless equity was specifically and purposely designed in, instead of just trying to reduce health disparities retroactively, the outcome would always be inequity. She pointed to several missed opportunities in this aspect throughout the pandemic, including issues such as scarce resource allocation (e.g., vaccines) (Parker et al., 2021) and hospital transfer issues within a region (Schorsch, 2020) while trying to maintain equitable care.

Staffing Considerations and Clinical Issues

Highlighting the multidisciplinary nature of hospital staffing, Anuj Mehta, assistant professor at the University of Colorado, emphasized the importance of the team-based mentality, saying it is at the core of their work in the hospital (see Figure 2-3). He elaborated on lessons learned regarding staffing and how it is interrelated with CSC planning and needs. While the focus in the media is often on the "stuff" that is in shortage, such as how to decide who gets limited ventilators, who gets beds, or who gets the limited oxygen supply, Mehta explained that what is actually occurring is that systems may have all of those resources but not have enough clinicians to deliver that care. He also reminded the audience that this issue of a health care workforce shortage was not new, but COVID-19 has brought a spotlight to it, reinforcing that staff are a finite resource and not infinitely flexible. Mehta noted that politicians talk about how staff can be stretched thinner, but eventually it does affect patient safety and morale in the field, with recent reports of 30 percent of health care workers considering leaving the field (Wan, 2021). This is truly an imminent crisis, he added.

Mehta also discussed various methods to augment the staffing crisis, but because trained workers are truly a finite resource, there is always a conse-

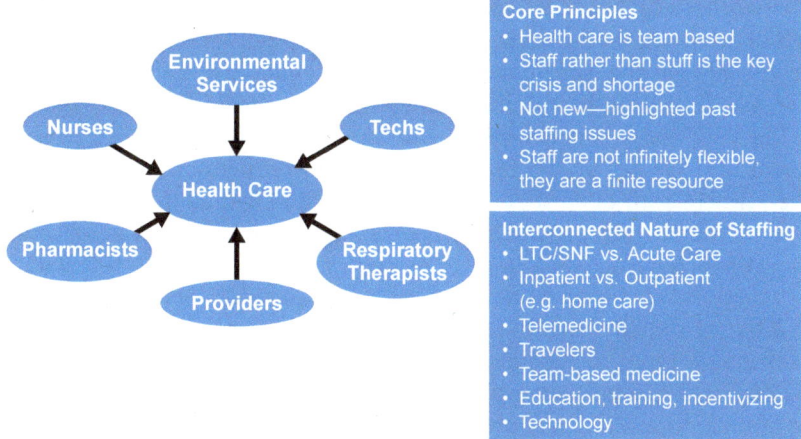

FIGURE 2-3 Core principles of multidisciplinary staffing in a hospital system.
NOTE: LTC/SNF = long-term care or skilled nursing facility.
SOURCE: Anuj Mehta presentation, September 27, 2021.

quence to most of the changes. For example, nurses and ancillary staff have moved from nursing homes and long-term care centers to acute hospitals and health care facilities to help with the increased surge of patients during the pandemic, creating a workforce shortage in nursing homes. This then makes it difficult for hospitals to offload patients who are ready to recover, so bed availability is still a challenge. But there are tweaks and process changes that can be employed to use technology and augment staffing, he noted. For example, in his ICU in Denver, they moved the patient's medication pump outside the room, so the respiratory therapist or nurses do not need to suit up in personal protective equipment every time they need to modify levels. This makes it easier for providers to care for multiple patients. But once the pandemic has truly ended or become much less of a threat, he concluded, hospitals and hospital systems need to think about how to augment staff, whether through new staffing models or other changes, so that the health care system can be more prepared for the next pandemic.

Mehta also provided an overview on the planning, implementation, and monitoring of CSC, highlighting several of the lessons that he has learned throughout the process. One of the key lessons he noted through the precrisis planning process in Colorado was the idea of community engagement. Often this is done as an afterthought, or just using feedback from doctors and lawyers involved in the absence of community, he said. But while rewriting the Colorado CSC plan, they met with people in an ongoing manner over several weeks, which contributed a large amount of helpful information regarding age-based and disability-based discrimination.

Another important lesson to consider during preplanning is the inclusion of equity in load-balancing[3] considerations across hospitals to ensure that people get the same care regardless of which hospital they are taken to. Crisis activation has been extremely variable throughout the pandemic, Mehta said, and what is on paper may be different than what is happening in real life. He advocated for more attention on defining certain triggers when either "staff or stuff" is in shortage. He highlighted the importance of determining how the process of triage is implemented ahead of time—all the way from activation, who constitutes the triage teams, how to calculate triage scores, how to reassess these scores, and how to triage transfer patients.

One of the challenges specifically with triage, he noted, is that there are different types to account for, not just multiple people waiting for one resource. For example, emergent triage relates to an unknown person coming into the hospital at any point, and it would be impossible to assess their needs ahead of time. But there is also prospective triage, where you are assessing survivability, but this also has nuances. Mehta shared that it can be quite difficult to weigh the needs of a person who shows up first versus the potential person who may come in later. It is also necessary to consider potential transfer patients.

Mehta said that as of September 2021, his ICU is not at a crisis activation level, but it does have patients from seven surrounding states and constantly receives calls from physicians in other states looking for beds. He noted there was also a need for monitoring and evaluation, but these are difficult to operationalize in a crisis. Other needs include monitoring before activation, and considering equity and fairness in the process, as well as reassessment. Reinforcing points made by Peek, he highlighted the need for having equity at the forefront of how planners are thinking about this process. As a final point, Mehta emphasized the importance of precrisis planning and exercising. He noted that while most CSC plans likely have triage teams enshrined in their process, it is necessary to have them practice and get a sense for the large moral burden they will endure by making some of these life-or-death decisions for people. He found this was an issue even just in a simulated exercise and recommended being aware of the mental health consequences and having the right resources available for staff.

Legal Lessons and Accountability

Jennifer Piatt, deputy director for the Network for Public Health Law–Western Region Office, offered lessons related to legal issues throughout the

---

[3] Load-balancing activities may include prehospital distribution of patients in other healthcare facilities in the area, patients transfers between facilities, or sharing resources between different facilities.

past decade of work. One of the first legal lessons highlighted in the 2019 workshop *Crisis Standards of Care: Ten Years of Successes and Challenges*,[4] she said, is that while the initial conception of triggers included express or formal state-based invocation of CSC plans, planners and hospital systems should be conceiving of CSC triggers much more broadly. This could be informed by federal guidance, existing CSC plans, or regional agreements. Emergency declarations can also help facilitate CSC implementation. This is important, she continued, because full or express political support for CSC at the state level may be lacking, leaving decisions to individual localities or health systems. Shortages can also occur in the absence, delay, or rescission of formal declarations, so systems should understand how to proceed without that type of support and establish consistency across jurisdictions.

A second lesson that was brought forward in the 2019 workshop and further highlighted during the COVID-19 experience is that of accountability and the existing patchwork of liability protections. Litigation has already begun to emerge in nursing facilities alleging negligence in some cases during the COVID-19 pandemic. Piatt added that it will be important to guarantee that adequate liability protections are in place to ensure that health care workers remain willing and able to provide services in crisis scenarios, but that it is also important not to go too far in that direction, and maintain levels of accountability by not protecting actions that are willful.

Piatt concluded that one of the most important issues that emerged in this process of operationalization was equity. HHS and other health authorities uncovered that many plans had built in age or disability discriminations in terms of how they were allocating resources. Over the course of the pandemic, the Office of Civil Rights (OCR) within HHS laid out guidance with green, yellow, and red light distinctions for how plans should be put together to avoid explicit discrimination (HHS, 2021). For example, sequential organ failure assessment (SOFA) scores have been found to adversely affect black patients, so discontinuing use of those as a scoring mechanism is an important lesson.

Discussion

Hanfling highlighted some of the points throughout the panel's presentations, noting that it is clear equity needs to be at the center of discussions, and providers need to remember to put the patient first in decisions. He reiterated Mehta's points on staffing, adding that the next iteration of CSC planning will need that level of detail and should focus on separating what

---

[4] https://www.nap.edu/catalog/25767/crisis-standards-of-care-ten-years-of-successes-and-challenges.

works from what does not, collecting the best practices that can be more widely applied.

Toner asked what could be done to improve situational awareness of the triggers, pointing out that many providers in the summer of 2021 knew that the Delta variant was outcompeting the Alpha variant in most regions, but all of their data and protocols were based on the Alpha variant. Hanfling replied saying there is a need to better hone data acquisition and increase the ability to examine data in real-time. He added that just 1 year ago, HHS did not have visibility on bed availability for tracking COVID-19 patients. In the midst of the emergency, it had to find a private company to help. This is an example of where more coordination at the federal level can help to provide interoperable systems.

Hanfling also saw an opportunity for health care coalitions to play a role in bringing information up from the local level. He noted that the goal of CSC planning is to have situational awareness driving decision making to avoid having to ration care. Mehta added that too often bed capacity is represented as physical beds, but "staffed beds" should be the critical measure, and that number is in flux every day. He also called for identifying an upper limit of what providers can handle and defining capacity during surges to ensure safety is prioritized.

Peek explained that in addition to aligning staffing with bed capacity and other resources, the quality of training that people get in tertiary care hospitals and community hospitals is variable. For example, a well-trained ICU physician can staff more beds than a different type of clinician. There needs to be a better understanding of what the true capacity is of available staff, she said, especially those serving communities who bear a larger burden of diseases and have higher proportions of COVID-19 patients. Finally, Vanderwagen added that the linkage between public health authorities and hospital facilities is very weak in most places, but there is a need to incentivize stronger dialogue between these sectors.

On triage and protocols, Mehta noted that SOFA is part of many triage protocols, but it was not designed for this level and scale of use. As of September 2021, there was still a poor understanding of who was likely to survive COVID-19, he said, as well as poor metrics. As another note on equity, Peek added that different social identities intersect in different ways and can affect equity. For example, thinking about race and age, she said, potential policies that have a strict age guideline must be considered within the context that not everyone might be able to get to that age. She explained that because of structural inequities, black people on average do not live as long compared to white populations. So, to make these concepts fairly accessible to everyone, protocols may need to be adjusted for these factors and must incorporate multiple types of vulnerability, she said.

Mehta added that triage for a ventilator, ICU bed, hospital bed, or dialysis all rest on different predictors. And there is no one singular algorithm that will satisfy the needs of saving the most lives while still being equitable. He said that core ethical principles by which health care professionals want to make those decisions must be defined, and real-time access to data is necessary to constantly be able to better inform the dynamic situation and needs. Hanfling added that federal government partners need to engage in this discussion to help advance to the next level of planning and capabilities. The best capabilities science can bring are needed to discover how to make smarter decisions, he said. For example, it is still unclear what the correlates of protection are for medical countermeasures, whether for COVID-19 or other risks.

In conclusion, Toner commented on how complex CSC truly is, and how many layers have emerged and continue to emerge from the COVID-19 pandemic, creating more need for learning. As of September 2021, this coronavirus, SARS-CoV-2, was only 5 percent as lethal as severe acute respiratory syndrome (SARS), which emerged in 2003, and 2.5 percent as lethal as Middle East respiratory syndrome (MERS), affecting multiple countries since 2015; the need for robust and engaged CSC planning is even more critical now than we thought it was in 2009, he stated.

3

Considerations for Staffing, Effects on the Workforce, and Future Trends

As Mehta mentioned earlier in the workshop series, while many traditionally consider "stuff" to be the limited resource within health care, such as oxygen, ventilators, blood, or drugs, it is often "staff" shortages that cause issues and lead to considerations for shifting to contingency or crisis standards of care (CSC) modes. Staffing shortages and their accompanying challenges have been encountered throughout the pandemic across sectors, making this notion painfully clear. In this chapter, the speakers highlight some of the key staffing challenges encountered throughout the COVID-19 pandemic, discuss specific issues with nurses and emergency medical services (EMS) personnel, and present potential short- and long-term solutions and best practices that have been employed over the last few years to attempt to mitigate some of the staffing shortfalls felt in various areas. Speakers discussed some of the changes enacted through emergency measures that should remain even after the crisis ends. Finally, invited speakers reflected on the ongoing nursing crisis in particular and discussed ways to improve the profession for the future.

EFFECTS OF COVID-19 ON THE WORKFORCE

Asha Devereaux, senior medical officer, Sharp Coronado Hospital, highlighted first responders, nurses, and doctors as the key stakeholders for the discussion. She shared a disaster response framework showing the continuum of care from conventional to contingency to crisis (see Figure 3-1).

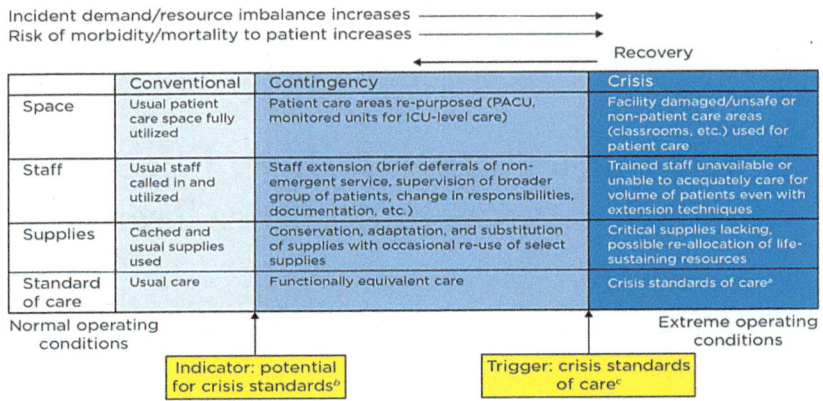

FIGURE 3-1 Disaster response framework for crisis standards of care.
SOURCE: Asha Devereaux presentation, October 11, 2021.

The original developers of this CSC framework envisioned indicators between the conventional and contingency phases that would help determine when the change was coming, and then triggers to know when to shift into crisis phase. This is not what happens in reality, she said. Instead, the lines are much more blurred and uncertain. Devereaux noted that even before the pandemic, there were staffing shortages, antiquated hiring and staffing mechanisms, a failure to view nurses as key talent within an organization, scope-of-practice policies lacking flexibility, and unusual payment structures financing the nursing workforce. The speakers discussed some of these issues and their contribution to staffing challenges in a crisis.

The Consequences of Moral Injury

Intuitively, there are many lessons learned, from many events, on how to move into CSC and how to address those crises, said Jeanette Ives Erickson, chief nurse emerita, Massachusetts General Hospital. Painting a picture of the country in February 2020, Erickson said, "We didn't know what we didn't know." However, pretty quickly, many ancillary services or nonessential surgeries and care delivery were cancelled, and those health workers found themselves thrown into an emergency response with varying levels of training. She concluded that the concept of intact teams was lost. She echoed Devereaux's concerns about the workforce shortages that existed even before the pandemic and said that now there is a projected worldwide shortfall of 18 million health workers by 2030, mostly in low- and lower-middle income countries (WHO, n.d.).

She reviewed some of the current issues with the health care workforce, noting that 30 percent are considering leaving their profession, and nearly 60 percent reported experiencing negative effects on their mental health as a result of their work throughout the pandemic (Kirzinger et al., 2021). Erickson emphasized that it is imperative that clinician burnout be given more attention as many of them have become cynical, exhausted, and have little sense of personal accomplishment this long into the pandemic. What is needed in this current moment, she said, is the courage to push on behalf of the workforce to build new systems and structures and invest in people. Erickson concluded that the real worry is about people in general and their moral distress and suffering, and that this is the bigger issue that demands attention.

Staffing Challenges across Sectors

Cynda Hylton Rushton, professor of clinical ethics, School of Nursing at Johns Hopkins University, built on Erickson's presentation, referencing the importance of the moral burden for the health care workforce. If you are the person deciding which person is seen first and who needs care the most, in an emergency room full of patients who need care, knowing that your decisions may likely cause harm to someone, it weighs heavily on you, she said, and it can lead to an accumulation of moral residue and suffering. She added that the pandemic has made this issue a chronic and unrelenting experience, a corrosive form of moral suffering, not just an episodic issue when there is a busy day. Rushton reported that 32 percent of clinicians and 38 percent of nurses had clinically significant symptoms of moral injury, showing how pervasive these consequences are (Rushton et al., 2021). She explained that moral injury is associated with posttraumatic stress disorder, increased depression, medical errors, and suicidal thoughts, creating another layered burden for clinicians, in addition to physical and psychological exhaustion.

While she appreciated the difficulty in distinguishing between the different standards of care, Rushton said that most clinicians have been operating in the contingency phase. But lacking regulatory and legal protections, they have been left to make individual allocation decisions without the benefit of a triage team or guidelines about how to resolve difficult ethical questions. She noted that this piece has been missing from this effort. She recalled her own time spent creating elegant allocation schemes for ventilators, blood, and drugs but realized they did not put the same effort into navigating the best ways to allocate human resources.

In the United States there are roughly one million EMS clinicians working in EMS agencies, said Gamunu Wijetunge, EMS specialist, Office of EMS, National Highway Traffic Safety Administration. In the course of

1 year, they typically respond to about 40 million events and 9-1-1 calls. Prior to the pandemic, it was common for clinicians to work at multiple positions, but this practice expanded during COVID-19 with clinicians working at many different locations, which has resulted in a strain on the 9-1-1 portion of EMS. In 2009, HHS led a nationwide assessment of state pandemic plans, revealing that there was no real planning for treatment of patients without transporting them to the hospital (HHS, 2009). Wijetunge explained that in his opinion, this was largely owing to reimbursement policy dating back decades, and that laws and regulations did not allow for "treat and refer."

Andrew Garrett, associate professor at George Washington University's School for Medicine and Health Sciences and senior advisor at the Office of the Assistant Secretary for Preparedness and Response (ASPR) at HHS, commented that the typical surge staffing model relied on by health care in most disasters has been a source of constraint in the pandemic. He highlighted two main practices within the model, saying often times the workforce just works harder and faster to get through it, thinking it will only last days or weeks, and then if that does not work, they borrow resources from other sources. Both of these practices have become problematic during a long-term pandemic, whether talking about personnel at a local hospital level or regional or state trade of an EMS compact. He explained that the pandemic has broken this all-hazards model that has worked fairly well up until now, and it has become clear that novel solutions, beyond those in the normal repertoire, are now needed.

Garrett said that workers cannot just work harder and faster to get it done; instead, we need to reimagine how crises and disasters are thought about and planned for in the United States, moving away from the short-term, high-impact disasters and shifting toward longer, more drawn out public health crises. Additionally, on top of the demands of 2020 and the pandemic, the rest of the world did not go away, Garrett noted. The year 2020 saw many large hurricanes that were added to the pandemic challenges, and staff and resources that would typically be needed for those responses became even more difficult to access and strained systems to the breaking point (Garrett, 2020).

Coming off of another week in the ICU at his hospital, Ryan Maves, professor of infectious disease, Wake Forest School of Medicine, said that stepping back as an attending physician and looking at the workforce implications of the current situation, he found two things most striking. The first was team cohesion, as there have been lots of shifts in where providers work and a lot of nurses moving because of travel agency work. As a result, he said there is a lack of continuity in busier hospitals, so every day it seems like you are working with a new team. He stated that one of the strengths of working in critical care typically is the mutual trust among everyone on the team. You know what each person's strengths are, and you know you can depend on them in stressful situations But with the current situation, care teams are meeting new people every day, and that mutual trust is lost. It influences efficiency when, for example, staff are actively decompensating patients, because one provider may not know what a nurse on the team knows, or the intubating process might be different, and this is an ongoing challenge.

The second factor he found striking, also alluded to by Anuj Mehta, is not a lack of physical beds, but a lack of people to staff them. Everyone is shifting their scopes of practice to try and optimize the workforce and pushing patients out into wards under care of staff that would never normally be expected to manage this level of patient severity, he explained, and this has a real effect on patient safety. There are benefits, as the system adapts over time and people learn new skills, but while that is happening, it can be extremely disruptive to have providers running around in three places with ICU nurses also functioning in the emergency department. He pointed out that typically within an ICU there are multiple different stakeholders on the team responsible for different procedures and tasks that they specialize in. He explained that this flexibility is not available anymore, and the pool of people to draw from has become smaller and smaller. At what point does the word *disaster* no longer apply, Maves asked, and at what point does this just become the way the world works?

Implications of Overburdened Staff and Lack of Team Culture

After the speakers' remarks, Devereaux asked about the structural impediments to communication of strain or stress. For example, in Florida during the height of the surge, doctors had gag orders placed on them for asking for help, and clinicians have been fired for vocally calling for assistance. What are some challenges in this area? Rushton agreed it was certainly a problem, and while violence against health care workers was present before, it has only escalated during the pandemic. Health care work is interconnected with societal injustice and structural disadvantages, she said, and many people are angry and outraged at different things. Previously there was a level of safety at your workplace, but now, no one feels safe. Rushton shared that we may be seeing the erosion of societal trust. In her work, the most common theme around moral injury was broken trust and the sense of betrayal. For example, institutions say that there are resources for clinicians to address mental health issues, but there is a culture that is associated with stigma and shame for those clinicians to admit that they need help.

Erickson added to the discussion about the lack of team cohesion by explaining that the continuous movement of staff between various clinical settings and between various teams leads to questions of safety. She pondered on how best to respond to the moment while ensuring the health care workforce remains safe. She pointed to the importance of taking a pause and getting back to the basic principle of human connection, and added that safety huddles throughout the day should be built into the structures and routine practices for care delivery.

Prior to the pandemic, there was an increasing focus on safety culture within EMS, said Wijetunge. He noted the ongoing need brought about by the pandemic to be more people centered and team centered, so patient and provider safety as well as mental health issues are being prioritized. More broadly, he added that one of the lessons learned is the critical need for more cross-sector collaboration, so EMS, public health, health care, and emergency management are all working closely together, with the challenges clearly outlined. Garret agreed that the health care system was thought of as much more integrated than it truly is, and existing fractures became highly magnified when the pandemic began.

There are cultural barriers to discussing the problems in EMS, said Garrett. He explained that typically an ambulance picks up a patient and drops them off at the hospital, and that the system evolved that way because of how these services are paid for in the United States. He added that if these everyday problems cannot be fixed, it will be difficult to implement even better models when there is a disaster. He suggested reimagining what the health care system looks like, from prehospital integrated health care to all specialties, with a "one coordinated fight" kind of approach to dealing with these major national catastrophes.

Devereaux asked about the lack of disaster preparedness and how that contributes to moral injury. Maves responded that the notion of triage is something that is well trained for in the military, and in that context people understand that in situations of austere resources, the priority should be to achieve the greatest good for the greatest number of people. However, this concept has only been in the civilian world for the last 18 months with constant triaging in health care. Maves believed that the pandemic opened up a window where the health care workforce can be trained in the concept of resource limitation, integrating it into a better appreciation for palliative care. He added that despite the circumstances, it is important to understand that even CSC are "standards of care," and there is always an ability to provide some care.

He noted that although health care workers always want to do more, it is important for them to accept that sometimes a certain level of care is what is available. He acknowledged that education will help better prepare providers for these decisions, but it will not be sufficient to remove the moral burden, and it will take a long time for the clinical community to get used to this idea. Rushton agreed that the moral burden will not be erased and that there is a need to better understand how to help people carry it without so much cost to themselves. She concluded that the process needed to be rehumanized and the focus shifted towards what is needed to better support both the people being cared for and those providing care.

PROMISING STAFFING STRATEGIES AND FUTURE DIRECTIONS

Lisa Rowen, chief nurse executive, University of Maryland Medical System, highlighted key strategies for managing staffing and workforce challenges across three time frames: today (immediate), short term (1–3 months), and longer term (greater than 3 months) (see Figure 3-2).

She suggested using technology for inpatient observation, such as tele-observation, instead of having a human observing the patient for safety. She explained this would allow for a more optimal use of both nurses and certified nurse assistants, because they do not have to stay in one room and deal with donning and doffing of personal protective equipment (PPE). She noted that staffing strategies have been the same for decades across the country; there are opportunities to streamline and optimize documentation and to deliver care so that it provides for and supports staff so they can gain time back in their day. There are also opportunities to create innovative roles, such as a "mobility tech," that can be filled by exercise physiology graduates who are interested in the work instead of certified nursing assistants, who are often difficult to recruit. Finally, for long-term strategies, she shared that providers can optimize how they order care and treatment to avoid lengthening the time nurses spend providing that care and treatment. Additionally, some providers are creating an integrated, innovative model

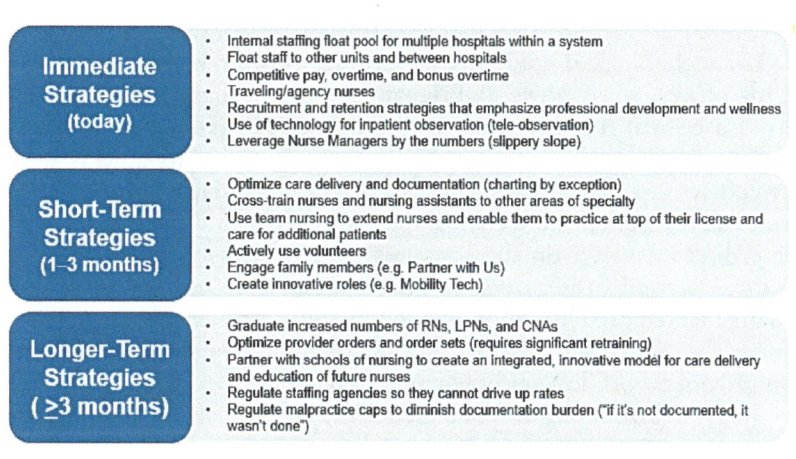

FIGURE 3-2 Current and potential solutions to staffing and workforce challenges.
SOURCE: Lisa Rowen presentation, October 11, 2021.

for care delivery and education by partnering with schools of nursing to align their clinical setting with the new education standards.

California completed its CSC concept of operations in 2020 after being put on hold, said Howard Backer, medical director, California Medical Assistance Teams, California EMSA, and the state turned out to be a miniature model of the country given the variety of surge needs and outcomes during COVID-19. He reported three main areas of managing surge: regulatory support, surge missions, and staffing models. All the interventions had an effect on staffing, whether they were direct or indirect.

The first step to manage surge is through regulatory support, he said, including declarations and regulatory or executive orders that may come from the governor, health officer, or EMS director in a state. Examples of this include expanded nurse–patient ratios, expanded scope of practice for EMS, licensing for retired or out-of-state providers, and a vaccine mandate for health care workers. Next, he explained, they had multiple surge missions that affected hospitals, such as through skilled nursing facilities support, alternate care sites, and load balancing across institutions, which was often challenging because of the amount of high-flow oxygen that ambulances needed to carry to support patients during transport. Finally, he reviewed some of their staffing models for this support, which included California's Disaster Medical Assistance Teams, which were highly mobile and flexible, as well as the National Guard, students, and retired personnel. He concluded by stating that this range of strategies used in California is what allowed them to stay out of the CSC phase, though he acknowledged they did go right up to the threshold of entering CSC.

Using Technology for Staffing

For technological solutions to staffing, Alistair Erskine, chief digital health officer, Mass General Brigham Hospital, shared that technology played a critical role across all environments of Mass General. Even for phone and online chat options, his hospital was able to quickly develop low-code or no-code algorithms, which could be adapted throughout the day, to advise patients and change the route of care and where people were being directed based on the hospitals' staffing capacities and bed availability. A second strategy was to have patients help, using patient portals and augmented capacity to be able to schedule visits using online tools and remove the burden from phone calls by embedding the virtual visits directly into provider workflow and the patient portal.

To avoid hospitalization of patients, the hospital also had virtual observation units where patients who typically would have been admitted were discharged home with a pulse oximeter and monitored virtually by staff. For acute care interventions, Erskine said that after ICUs were overwhelmed in Boston during the first wave, staff realized the solution was to form a virtual ICU. The hospital needed a dashboard for ICU awareness, so Erskine's staff virtualized the consultation of the ICU doctor and remote monitoring across the hospital system. Medical isolation was also an important issue to overcome, so the hospital purchased tablets for every hospitalized patient and converted rooms to video and audio, which, similar to Rowen's strategies, saved nursing time in donning and doffing PPE.

Staffing shortages in medical surgery led to making virtual rounds, so there was a much smaller team in hospital, he explained. But this way, even staff who had been exposed and needed to be quarantined could still work remotely and safely write notes and place orders. The hospital also needed to conduct COVID-19 testing and vaccinations for staff, so a portal was created for employees that included daily scheduling of testing and shots and another dashboard was created for staff awareness. This also included a mental health app to support staff.

One thing that was missing, Erskine noted, was a scalable, automated communication strategy for patients, as the outreach for patients missed the opportunity to gather responses from them about their treatment. They tried to manually identify high-risk patients to prioritize invitations to schedule a COVID-19 test or vaccination but realized that using the EMR transactional system to do so was very work intensive. A consumer relationship management tool that many retail organizations use could do this in a much more efficient and streamlined way, he said, so they are now in the process of creating that.

Supporting Health Care Workers

Alexander Niven, associate professor in pulmonary and critical care medicine at the Mayo Clinic, proposed potential solutions to the epidemic of burnout in health care workers that has occurred since March 2020. It is important to highlight the balance between resilience and workplace stressors, he said, as this was tilted in the wrong direction even prior to the pandemic. This imbalance is forcing health care workers into situations where they are regularly engaging in nonfunctional overreaching, which translates to increased burnout and errors. An important part of the conversation that is often left out are the stabilizing influences that can come from the quantity and quality of work, Niven explained, and the influences of cultural support within teams and health care organizations. Those elements are out of individuals' direct control, and the scope goes beyond the individual. If left unaddressed, he underlined the potential damage to care that is delivered to patients and the potential damage done to the system in terms of lower-quality care, medical errors, decreased productivity, and increased turnover and costs (see Figure 3-3).

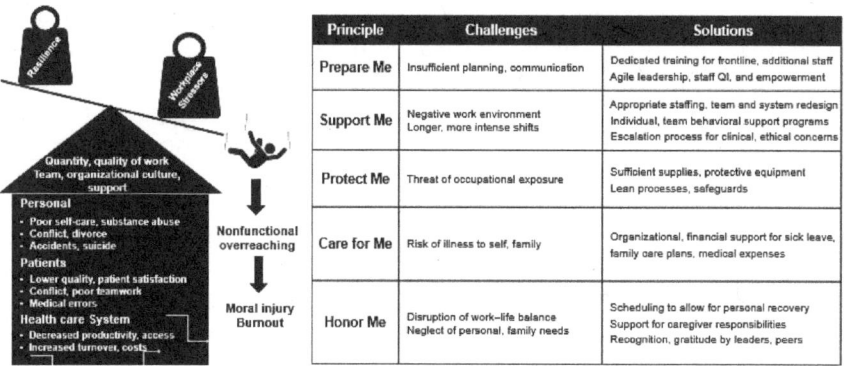

FIGURE 3-3 Prevention, mitigation of moral injury, and burnout in health care workers during times of crisis.
SOURCE: Alexander Niven presentation, October 11, 2021.

All of these ramifications underline the moral imperative that needs to be added to this existing dashboard for the learning health care system to improve, stated Niven. Dashboards already exist to look at safety, quality, cost, and performance on a regular basis; adding validated measures for staff burnout to that dashboard and monitoring it regularly would require marginal additional commitments. Also displayed in Figure 3-3, Niven shared some challenges and solutions based on a series of interprofessional focus groups conducted by Stanford University early in the pandemic. People are able to focus on delivering high-quality care when they do not have to worry about their own safety and security, Niven said. Creating organizational support structures that include sick leave, family care plans, caregiver assistance, and allowing a scheduling system that does allow for recovery can significantly help mitigate staff burnout.

Discussion on Structural Impediments to Staffing

While some have proposed increasing the number of new nurses and graduates as a solution to these challenges, a participant asked if these new recruits are just being put into the same environment that is causing current staff to leave. Rowen responded that the biggest reason staff are feeling burned out and demoralized is the lack of staff and other team members to share the burden of patient care. Nursing is typically a 90 percent female workforce, and 70 percent of them have either children or parents they are caring for, with the COVID-19 crisis amplifying those needs. Rowen added that she believes the travel nurse industry greatly reduced the number of nurses available to staff hospitals and clinics, in part because those agencies were able to offer elevated pay rates, as high as $275/hour (salaried nurses would make two-thirds of that), and it became difficult for hospitals and health care centers to retain their staff and compete with these rates. However, she does believe that graduating more nurses and putting them in acute care settings will rebalance the equation, because the need for travel nurses lessens and more nurses will be in positions at the bedside. Early in the pandemic, Devereaux noted that many providers were furloughed or sidelined from work, which is what contributed to increased numbers in these alternate agencies or workforces.

Highlighting a related question, Devereaux asked if the health care workforce is lumped in as a resource, like a ventilator, that can be driven into CSC. She asked whether it was the right way to think about staff. Niven responded that humans are more than just a resource. He reiterated the importance of interpersonal relationships and shared his experience in creating a high-performing health care team. These concepts cross the gap between the bedside and the digital environment being created. He stated that human beings are naturally going to look for personal security and family security first, which are reasonable core values and should be considered by health systems if they want to retain a highly skilled and seasoned workforce. Without that, he continued, there will be a loss of manpower and constant turnover and staff churn, which degrades overall workflow and quality. Erskine added that those health care workers will need to adapt to the technology system and system of care, which involves training and electronic learning to bring the person up to speed, and this will take additional time and effort.

Devereaux asked how funding has become a challenge for staffing solutions and what the concerns might be. Rowen responded that paying high rates for certain services, like travel nursing, takes money away from what we can do about pay rates and benefits for internal staff. Hospitals are directing a huge amount of funding toward this temporary, mobile workforce instead of investing in loyal workers, committed to an institution, she continued. Backer added that in California there have been several mentions about the importance of highly functional teams. While this is easier to do with long-term staff, in a disaster you have to be more creative and bring in staff from many different sources—sometimes blending national, state, local, and occasionally military backgrounds. He added this may need to become a part of normal daily options for health care systems.

Health care is under stress at the best of times, and it could just take a bad flu season to use all the resources of a hospital and require tents and additional surge staffing. The State of California found that during the first few waves of COVID-19, the state covered all the costs for staffing. When the state tried to wean recipients off of state funding and send them to contract agencies to maintain the added capacity, he noted there was a lot of resistance, so it had to be a very gradual process. Another point of response is that there were different compositions of teams, and Backer said EMS personnel are a good way of supplementing health care teams because they are flexible. Backer concluded that paramedics cannot replace nurses but they complement them quite well in an acute care setting. But once a hospital changes back from crisis and contingency to standard conventional care, then often the regulation exemptions and the territoriality of professional societies and unions returns and brings challenges to the mixed staffing models.

Emergency Changes That Should Become Standard

Devereaux raised another question: which of the changes seen recently in health care should remain permanent? Rowen replied that during the crisis hospitals changed what was required for documentation and charting and moved to exceptions for charting. Clinicians then assumed things were okay unless it was documented that something was not done. This change flipped how we document, she said, and it actually saves a lot of time, so we are now moving toward making this our standard practice. Erskine added that patient expectation also changed significantly regarding virtual care. There is no putting the "genie back in the bottle." Knowing the level of convenience and reduced costs that come with virtual care, he predicted that this trend will likely persist. But there may need to be ongoing legislation about what can and cannot be done. Erskine noted that this idea was taken from the retail industry and applied appropriately in the health care space to let patients self-serve and have health care become less of a black box, while making providers more available at the patient's schedule. This is a good change that should persist, he added.

Niven stated that from his standpoint, his organization broke down many siloes regarding staffing individual work areas and was able to maximize capacity and capabilities both within and outside the organization. His organization also recognized, especially in COVID-19 ICUs, that bedside care with PPE demands was extremely difficult, so it used the increased demand for electronic health resources as an opportunity to rotate staff and expand the pool of workers who can engage in those services to give them a break from the extremely burdensome PPE. Backer added that the long-term nature of this response has ingrained the emergency management concepts and practices deeply into the health care system. Not only do health systems and facilities know how to go into emergency mode and request resources, he said, but the process has become more embedded into common knowledge. Rowen also noted that her organization focused on team member wellness throughout the past 20 months, which has been appreciated. Management and leadership teams were prioritized, and this

REFLECTIONS ON THE NURSING CRISIS AND FUTURE DIRECTIONS

Tener Goodwin Veenema, contributing scholar and professor of nursing at Johns Hopkins Center for Health Security, presented some final reflections on the current nursing crisis throughout the country. The most dangerous thing that can be done, she argued, is to go back to normal and business as usual. She called for transformational change to create and sustain safer and more supportive workplace settings. This should include taking care of employees and humanizing workplace settings, designing systems to treat people with respect and value, and build the trust needed in order to build those trusted teams. Health care systems, hospitals, and other settings need to acknowledge nurses as talent, she said, just like any other workforce that needs to be recruited, developed, and maintained. She listed various ideas to improve the crisis, shown in Box 3-1.

BOX 3-1
Suggestions to Improve the Nursing Crisis

- Seek transformational change to create and sustain safe supportive workplace settings.
- Acknowledge nurses as talent that must be recruited, developed, and retained within health care organizations.
- Address the perverse payment structures that finance the nursing workforce.
- Overhaul human resource policies and programs to support diversity, equity, and inclusion.
- Eliminate barriers that constrain staff mobilization and deployment.
- Invest in nursing in ways that promote the health of women in the workplace.
- Promote career development plans for nurses.
- Improve elasticity in hospital staffing models in order to pivot quickly to reassign nurses as needed.
- Appreciate the time and investment needed to educate and train a critical care nurse (eliminate the "a nurse is a nurse" concept).
- Bring nursing care delivery up to date, including telenursing and e-ICU.
- Implement plans to achieve load balancing of nursing staff across health systems or regions.
- Increase nurse preparedness and their understanding of crisis standards of care.

SOURCE: Presented by Tener Goodwin Veenema.

COVID-19 has reopened old wounds in terms of professional hierarchies and lack of a voice within nursing, Veenema stated. She added that the value of nursing has long been obscured by hospital accounting practices that treat nurses more as undifferentiated labor costs. Additionally, while many traveling nurses are very committed and put their own health at risk in order to work, that system is adversely affecting the nursing workforce overall. She pointed to the existence of perverse payment structures that perpetuate this fragmented and disjointed system and concluded that there was a need to investigate how the nurses of this country can be better served.

In terms of understanding moral injury and supporting health care workers, Niven highlighted a final gap: there is no data regarding respiratory therapists, EMTs, or other allied health workers. That is something that needs to be understood and measured if solutions are to be found. Erskine added that people have realized health care is very labor dependent, but there are some places and processes that are amenable to technological solutions. It is incumbent on us to understand which aspects can be automated and how to share in decision making to augment care, he explained. Rowen added that there is a duty to partner with schools, whether nursing, medicine, or others, and "do it differently." As students and interns are integrated into clinical settings, the model of care needs to be morphed into something different and more sustainable, she said, so students get a better bedside education and current staff get better support within various settings. Backer added that even the best facilities and hard infrastructure cannot provide health care without staff. While equipment and ventilators can be shifted around easily, staff cannot, and it remains the number one needed element, he said.

4

Crisis Standards of Care: From Plans to Reality

While some institutions, cities, and states have been working on crisis standards of care (CSC) plans for several years, most of those efforts have been holding theoretical exercises and hosting community engagement discussions about hypothetical scenarios. Taking written plans and guidelines and putting them into practice during a true emergency is much less common for most jurisdictions. These instances are often when the key facets of a plan are best tested. In this chapter, speakers discussed various case studies of jurisdictions that have CSC plans and the lessons they learned in the process of creating those plans, especially relating to difficult tasks such as triage. This chapter also contains discussions on challenges related to workforce preparation, decision making, and public and stakeholder perceptions.

SETTING THE STAGE

Anuj Mehta, assistant professor of medicine, Denver Health and Hospital Authority, walked through the spectrum of changing needs from the conventional phase to the contingency phase to the crisis phrase and explained the different facets of CSC planning that need to occur in each phase. He explained that the conventional care phase, when there is no emergency, is when authorities and decision makers could identify the core principles on which they will be basing their decisions, as well as the key stakeholders to involve. As needs change and it looks like an emergency is imminent, other considerations include defining what supplies need to be triaged (i.e., what type of disease or emergency is it), who the triage team will consist of, and how those triage decisions will be made. Once the entity is operating in contingency mode with the potential to shift into crisis mode, he added, efforts move from purely planning to implementation. At this point, types of triage need to be defined, as well as the triggers or what it will take to activate CSC. Finally, Mehta said, once an institution is in crisis mode, there needs to be constant evaluation of equity implications of the protocols, ongoing assessment of data gathering and triage team processes, consideration of appeals, and deciding what will warrant deactivation of CSC.

John Hick, professor of emergency medicine, University of Minnesota, asked about supporting bedside clinicians for decision support, and Mehta noted that CSC does not just mean allocation of care. It could be altering dialysis time frames or putting two people into one room in an ICU. These processes or methods of disrupting care standards need to be identified early on, along with ethical principles that can guide decision making, Mehta said. Without an ethical foundation it will be difficult to ensure that factors unrelated to the patient and underlying disease are not influencing decisions. Mehta added that nonmedical sectors that rely on logistics, such as shipping companies and ride-share companies, know where all of their assets are at any point in time. He observed that health care is decades behind this and may need a better system for situational awareness and recognizing shifts throughout the day.

IMPLEMENTATION CASE STORIES

To provide varied perspectives on how CSC is implemented in different scenarios, this section provides experiences from three states across a range of planning needs, including community engagement, communication and coordination, and managing triage guidelines and workflows.

Incorporating Community Input in Colorado

Gina Febbraro, planning and improvement consultant, Colorado Department of Public Health and Environment (CDPHE), explained that while Colorado had been working on CSC plans when the pandemic began, concerns started to emerge from communities across the state. Many structurally marginalized communities were fearful of discrimination and implicit bias being embedded in the new CSC guidelines. CDPHE set up initiatives during the pandemic to engage communities and hear their equity concerns about what might be incorporated into guidelines. It is important for planners and providers to consider this process, Febbraro said, noting that it requires a different skill set to be able to engage the community in a meaningful way, especially those people who might not understand the complexity of CSC factors and plans. She highlighted the benefits of having a strong process and people who understand the principles of community engagement.

Describing the process Colorado undertook, Febbraro said her team recruited different community leaders and by the end of March 2020 was convening weekly group meetings and discussing the concerns and fears of each community at each meeting. Her team also developed a survey for community leaders that led to additional website resources being developed, and acknowledged the importance of these conversations both to influence policy and educate the public. She recalled the media highlighting the triaging of ventilators and ICU beds at the time, which is where her team had to focus much of their initial conversations.

Febbraro also remarked on some of the indirect results of this initiative, saying that relationships were formed and expanded beyond just CSC, and these relationships were able to inform other aspects of the entire response, including vaccine rollout at the state level. Some of the strengths of their process included diverse representation and the ability to be nimble, move quickly, and scale up as needed. Because the pandemic was ongoing and very present in people's lives—sometimes meaning life or death—she also commented that partners were very committed and engaged, which was a huge value. But limitations were also uncovered, such as structural racism being embedded in institutions. Government health care research and algorithms are integrated into CSC planning, so while these limitations were identified, it was difficult to tease out the areas of bias. Finally, Febbraro said that because of the rapid pace of the pandemic, the team had to move very quickly and were not able to use all the best practices of community engagement that would have been ideal during conventional planning phases.

Communication and Coordination in New Mexico

Chris Emory, chief of the Bureau of Health Emergency Management, New Mexico Department of Health, introduced New Mexico as a very large, primarily rural frontier state with very limited resources. He noted the state has one of the lowest number of hospital beds per capita in the country, so they have had to focus on coordination and communication between stakeholders across the state. As a state, New Mexico started CSC planning in 2018 after the Ebola outbreak, which resulted in a living document that was revised continually throughout the COVID-19 response. He explained that the initial planning team to create that document was given the Institute of Medicine CSC workbooks as well as a copy of Dr. Sheri Fink's book, *Five Days at Memorial,* to inform their process and set the groundwork for planning. They then held a full-scale exercise for pandemic influenza in 2018 that allowed for some testing of CSC plans and identifying the gaps in allocating resources across the state. It ended up also being an exercise where they focused on the need to practice "rational care versus rationing care." In other words, Emory said, they realized that within the state they had a critical need to develop transport capacity and transport pathways as well as surge capacity.

Once the pandemic emerged in early 2020, Emory said they had just finished revisions to the plan and knew they needed to build capacity to implement their plan. They followed a hub-and-spoke model, identifying three core hub facilities in the metro areas of Albuquerque and the regional hubs of Farmington, Santa Fe, Roswell, and Las Cruces to cover the four corners of the large state. These hospitals were selected based on their care capabilities as well as traditional transport pathways used in the state. Emory reported that those hospitals also were on the medical advisory team for the CSC plan, which was expanded during COVID-19. Throughout the response, the chief medical officers and chief operating officers from those facilities reached out to their spoke facilities daily or weekly to maintain their ongoing situational awareness of their needs and priorities, which was a great method for filtering information up to the state level.

They learned a lot throughout the process, making some initial mistakes, but Emory shared some successes as well, such as facilities being able to flex up to 150 percent of their license capacity. New Mexico also achieved statewide load balancing across facilities, had one central call center for the entire state, and maintained a constant continuum of care assessment, using space, staff, and supplies as core components to address the needs of various facilities.

Learning from COVID-19 in New York City

Elizabeth Chuang, Albert Einstein College of Medicine Montefiore Medical Center, focused her comments on the scarce resource triage component of CSC. Beginning in 2018, she conducted focus groups with key clinical stakeholders to solicit feedback on ventilator allocation draft policies and found that clinicians were worried about threats to their roles and identity, including decision making, autonomy, and fiduciary duty to the patient. While the team found their draft protocol to be necessary and acceptable, this early preparation was still challenged significantly by the emergence of COVID-19. The first barrier her team encountered was the lack of infrastructure to manage the implementation of potential triage protocols.

For example, at the time in early 2020, Chuang noted that the sequential organ failure assessment (SOFA) score was still used in many exemplar triage protocols, but in the first few weeks of the pandemic in New York

City, they were not able to obtain an automated SOFA score on patients with respiratory failure and had to calculate hundreds of scores by hand. They also lacked a reliable way to know how many ventilators were actually in use across the hospital system. These are common information infrastructure challenges across the country, she added. Additionally, while they were planning for potential implementation of triage protocols, they were tripling their ICU capacity, so support staff were busy working on those activities, making it difficult to prioritize triage operations.

Turning to workflows, Chuang noted that while guidelines had been available for years, tangible workflow plans, with appropriate levels of detail, were lacking. It was not clear how often the triage team should meet or how decisions would be made or communicated to teams and family members. Decisions also needed to be made about who would serve on the triage teams, since so many providers were desperately needed for direct patient care. There was also a lack of explicit support for public health expertise generally, and triage planning—specifically at the state government level—was a major obstacle to this planning work. It left hospitals uncertain whether triage protocols and workflows would be legitimized, and this disincentivized investment in these critical planning activities. She shared that through interviews with triage planners across the country, her team learned that states with supportive state governments had hospital leadership that was more willing to engage with triage planning and were able to conduct tabletop exercises to make the logistical steps of triage concrete and identify and correct workflow issues. Hospitals in the states without such support were less sure which activities would be sanctioned and had fear that press leaks of these activities would reflect poorly on the hospitals, making it difficult to complete the necessary training activities that would have allowed a smoother implementation.

In addition, the lack of national coordination led to scarcities of PPE, supplies, and medication that were unanticipated. Although her hospital never had to triage ventilators, Chuang said, other shortages required the rapid development of strategies for augmenting or allocating those resources. Given the difficulties of informing triage committees and workflows, Chuang noted the missed opportunity to bring together a formal team to manage difficult allocation decisions such as triaging the use of high-flow nasal cannula or providing fewer hours of dialysis to allow more patients access.

Finally, she highlighted the shortcomings of pre-COVID-19 triage guidelines, which are being documented more and more, such as the increasingly evident notion that SOFA scores are not appropriate for this use. Many concerns emerged from disability and minority communities, resulting in uncertainty and moral distress for those in positions of implementation planning, which was exacerbated by the lack of federal, state, and public support for these activities. She argued that in the future states should mandate preparedness activities and make resources available ahead of the next disaster in order to better navigate implementation of response activities. She concluded that implementation plans should also be transparent and public so debates on their legitimacy can take place ahead of a crisis.

Discussion

Hick asked for comments on the role of the triage team at a facility versus the regional level, and the best ways to make these roles consistent. Chuang said her medical center based its model on the Institute of Medicine CSC framework, and developed a triage committee internally, but more standardization across the region could be facilitated, especially with strong state government support. Tying in the hub-and-spoke model, Emory added that New Mexico's central call number has been critical from the standpoint of coordination. In an effort to address standardization across the state, they trained triage officers and those working in the call center to recognize and counter implicit biases. Most stakeholders do not know what CSC plans are, added Febbraro, so there is a job to do at the state level and in partnership with hospitals to continue the education of, and communication with, stakeholders and communities. Even though Colorado never had to activate its plan for triage for devices, she said a vast majority of their discussions with communities concerned the triage of ventilators and ICU beds and what would inform those decisions. The art of this community engagement is bringing diverse groups of people together and being able to speak openly about the principles and trade-offs that may be necessary.

Recalling the comments on moral distress for triage teams, Hick asked about how such distress plays out during exercises and real-world experiences, and how it affects the ability for institutions to operationalize these teams. Chuang responded that it is difficult to find people who recognize this is a real need that demands a system for operationalizing. These critical decisions should not be left to stressed bedside clinicians, she said, but it is also difficult to find people who want to engage in these discussions when there is not a crisis. She added that this type of work is challenging and not popular, and no one wants to add to that moral distress, so there is a need to incentivize it during noncrisis times to ensure it is addressed.

Load balancing across a state can work well until everything is full, noted Hick, and without some type of doubling up, things start to fall apart, and then it becomes very difficult to place patients. He asked whether there are policies in place that ensure fair access once everything is saturated. The first three waves of COVID-19 caused a greater focus on better coordination of transport in New Mexico, said Emory, but the current surge—of COVID-19 and other conditions—has reached the upper limit of state capacity. Data has been key throughout the response, and the state has been able to stay nimble and determine the critical resources needed, but the state had to declare CSC in October 2021 to provide additional protections through credentialing providers and allowing people to work outside their scope. Emory said they wrote a public health order allowing facilities to declare CSC at an individual facility level, based on lessons from previous waves. It is an ongoing effort, he noted, so it is difficult to say what is working well, but they are working within the hub-and-spoke model to ensure any available resource or space is being used efficiently. He said that right now New Mexico is getting to the point where the system is overly saturated.

While the flexibility of different facilities declaring CSC is nice, it can also lead to pockets of inconsistent or variable care, said Hick. Chuang reported that in New York, the state association helps to coordinate some of these processes to standardize approaches within a region. One area this would help is public trust, she added, so people know they are getting the same level of care regardless of the hospital they are taken to. Febbraro commented that this was a very difficult concept to communicate, because if the state made a CSC declaration, it did not bind hospitals to follow those guidelines; they had discretion to choose how they implemented them. The public often felt like the government at the state level should be able to hold hospitals accountable, but that is not the case. Instead, she suggested having open and honest conversations about how health departments and hospitals implement standards.

EXPLORING CHALLENGES IN CRISIS STANDARDS OF CARE

To highlight challenges from various perspectives, this section features views and opinions from different stakeholders regarding workforce preparation, decision making, and public perceptions regarding CSC.

Workforce Preparation

Emily Kidd, medical director for Acadian Ambulance in San Antonio, Texas, provided a local perspective on planning and implementation in a large EMS system in Texas. When it comes to numbers of disasters, Texas is number one, she said, so it has had many opportunities to think about CSC. For those hospitals still developing plans, she emphasized the importance of understanding the state laws and rules related to EMS and medical direction. Some states have an EMS medical director, but some—like Texas—do not, so EMS medical directors have to make decisions for their local agency without state oversight.

Kidd shared examples of medical director involvement in implementing CSC, such as outlining altered standards of care, and noted these are difficult decisions to make, choosing which patients will get which types of care, similar to the alterations made in an overrun hospital. Medical directors also had to change medications and treatments, especially early in the pandemic before the virus was well understood. Many EMS medical directors altered criteria for terminating resuscitation in the field, or not transporting patients to the hospital and just treating them in the field. Additionally, she explained, there were changes such as varying destinations for transport, altered dispatch protocols, and using EMS personnel in nontraditional roles (e.g., giving vaccines, working in monoclonal antibody centers). All of this has to be under the purview and protocols of the EMS medical director, Kidd stated, so it is important for them to be involved in all aspects of CSC planning well in advance of an emergency event.

Hick asked about the added burden on EMS of interfacility transfers during the pandemic, when there were often longer distances than usual that required additional coordination. Kidd agreed this was a critical issue, and though everyone thinks of 9-1-1 when they consider EMS, interfacility transport of patients is just as important. There were very long times for interfacility transport, she said, because full hospitals resulted in longer transport distances, or because EMS was overwhelmed or having staffing shortages. There is a need to balance having sufficient staff and ambulances to respond to 9-1-1 calls while also being able to complete hospital transfers, but this has been a significant challenge that will likely continue.

Erin Talati Paquette, assistant professor of pediatrics and School of Law at Northwestern University, shared challenges on the pediatric side throughout the pandemic. First, she noted the effect of the illness on pediatric patients and institutions, saying that although children in general have lower rates of infection and severe infection, they still needed to create the same triage preparation for pediatric institutions if the regional system was stressed to maximal capacity. What became challenging in this setting was that the use of ventilators and life-sustaining therapies in small children is not readily translatable to adults, so using the same criteria was not a good method.

There were some algorithms and protocols that had been in development for children that they tried to use to predict and triage supplies, but this proved quite a challenge, Paquette noted. Another consideration was how pediatric institutions can optimize their ability to serve as resources in a setting where there is an overall strain on the medical system. Many served as regional sites for consolidating pediatric care or increased their age eligibility to try and decompress adult facilities, but there were several barriers to consolidation—mirroring many of the adult challenges.

Within the pediatric workforce, Paquette said, there was a drive for providers wanting to work at the top of their license. But in terms of staffing plans, the desire for individuals to work with adults needed to be balanced with contingency planning in case there was a pediatric surge. It was also critical to ensure that individuals providing services would have adequate coverage if they became ill or had to quarantine. Regarding training, she said it is important to work on calibrating the workforce towards fluidity of resources—trying to have the same person serve in a variety of roles—but this requires coordination across multiple departments and services. Many pediatric providers were used to help with messaging and public health measure compliance, helping to create honest messaging about transmission and risk to children and vaccine hesitancy.

Paquette emphasized the need for coordination beyond one's own hospital system. Her system relied on the Chicago Bioethics Commission, a voluntary gathering in the Chicago area that worked on trying to have consistent guidelines across hospitals for adult and pediatric populations, she noted. Her system also tried to interface with local public health authorities and follow guidance from relevant associations, but it faced many of the same barriers in terms of communicating the changes in usual practices when trying to coordinate resources across regions and states. To truly have regional coordination, the authorities are important, concluded Paquette, because individual institutions cannot enact any kind of regional standardization, which makes it difficult when working across so many different facilities.

Decision Making

Brian Garibaldi, associate professor of medicine, Johns Hopkins Biocontainment Unit, introduced the general process his health system in Maryland used to approach the difficult decisions of allocating scarce resources. He first emphasized the goals of maximizing treatment benefit and enhancing survival, and any policy that is developed needs to be iterative and tested in an ongoing manner. Garibaldi also highlighted that there is no one correct approach, and decisions and principles will be different and individualized to each hospital or location. Thankfully, in his experience, Johns Hopkins did not have to allocate ventilators or ICU beds, but it did reach a point with therapeutics and extracorporeal membrane oxygenation machines.

When looking at its tools for ventilator allocation, Garibaldi's unit examined four different elements that underscored the prioritization of who would get a ventilator: short-term survival, long-term survival, clinical trajectory, and random chance. Because these elements could be subjective and variable, his team piloted a project where it created scarce resource allocation teams to examine patients who would be eligible, and had the providers score long-term survival. Garibaldi reported that the allocators did agree on whether someone made it one year or more after their current hospitalization (Ehmann et al., 2021).

When determining these policies, there were a number of outcomes his unit considered, Garibaldi said. The first was patient outcomes and trying to maximize treatment and survival, but he added that it was also important to have patient satisfaction and trust from the family and caregivers. The same is true for care providers, he said, since they were not making direct decisions about scarce resource allocation, but they needed to know the process was fair so they could trust the decisions.

From an organizational standpoint, Garibaldi explained his unit wanted to improve survival and quality of life but wanted to be sure it was maintaining trust and integrity with the community it served, so the community needed to be involved in the process in order to support it. He also reviewed the appeals process for patients and families, saying the process depends on the resource in question. If the decision was made not to offer mechanical ventilation to a patient and the patient wanted to appeal, the person would be given the treatment in question until the appeal could be considered by a special team. He highlighted the importance of testing how these appeals and processes work; his unit is retrospectively looking at COVID-19 patients and evaluating how the allocators and scores would have worked out looking at patient outcomes or potential alternatives. In real time, the reality is that people try the best they can, but now that there is so much data accumulated, he said, there is a need to think more carefully about identifying how the processes and methods for decision making can be improved.

Vikramjit Mukherjee, medical director of the Special Pathogens Program and director of the Medical ICU at Bellevue Hospital Center, shared his perspective from New York City, responding to the COVID-19 pandemic in spring 2020. Unfortunately, he said, most of the patients his hospital saw were those from traditionally underserved communities without good access to health care. He noted that there were mismatches in resources across the board, including staff, space, and supplies, which also took a toll on provider wellness. The effect of this on staff is still unresolved, Mukherjee added, and he expects posttraumatic stress disorder will stick with staff for years to come.

During the first surge, ICU beds filled quickly, he explained, so his ICU had to develop novel spaces or double up on patients in ICU rooms. He noted that while his team did not have to allocate ventilators, other elements of critical care medicine were often in short supply, so the resource mismatch was present across all domains. Unfortunately, he said, decision making was often arbitrary, as there was not clear guidance on who gets the state-of-the-art ventilators versus the old or borrowed ones, or who gets first-line therapy care versus other processes. He lamented that overall the processes and decisions resulted in some inequities.

Communication was another area that could be much improved, Mukherjee shared, as there should have been better communication with medical operation centers to provide situational awareness and information to the front lines. Working well across health systems was also a challenge, he noted, saying it was painful to see ICU beds totally empty 100 miles north, but New York City was on fire—there was no concept of load balancing. In conclusion, he emphasized that the space between conventional and crisis modes is when they try to do everything they can, coming up with all types of creative solutions to avoid reaching the critical point where resources are rationed. Hick highlighted the delicate balance between waiting too long to activate CSC and actually rationing the resource. Mukherjee agreed that it is a very careful line, but for something like dialysis, it makes more sense to offer half dialysis to 100 patients compared to full dialysis to just 50 patients. Having a clinical eye to inform many of the command center operations is critical in order to make these nuanced calls about resources, he stated.

Public and Stakeholder Perceptions

Julie Reiskin, executive director of the Colorado Cross-Disability Coalition, shared that she represents a community that is distrustful of both medicine and government, so when the pandemic emerged there were some immediate concerns. She highlighted what her coalition did in Colorado to gain community trust in the pandemic response. The historical experiences the people in the coalition have endured has created a perception, she explained, but when there is a significant event that engages community leaders, new perceptions can be formed. Reiskin noted that these changes happened when people at the health department invited leaders from the disability community to come to the meetings to be part of the discussions. As a result of that, changes were made to the CSC plans that removed many of the concerns for people within the disability coalition.

Explaining CSC and triage is hard, she said, as most people in this community have been told they will not survive something, so the concept of survivability causes suspicion. As a result, members of the coalition needed messaging in a way that was clear and not patronizing. One thing that built trust more than anything else, she said, was that people from the health department were willing to answer questions throughout the pandemic. She gave the example of a household in a rural community with two severely disabled people who were trying to navigate how to manage caregivers going in and out. Through these discussions, they had access to people who were knowledgeable and connected, and they were able to get the right PPE for the caregivers and follow the right public health measures, allowing trust to be built while those individuals stayed in their own home. Consequently, she shared that there was very little vaccine hesitancy in the disability community. Inviting community members in, listening to their concerns, and making changes where reasonable is critical for community trust, Reiskin concluded.

Elizabeth Lee Daugherty, chief wellness officer and associate professor of medicine at Johns Hopkins School of Medicine, shared a project from Maryland that was conducted, beginning in 2013, to better understand the issues in the community related to allocation of resources. Her team gathered participants from the community and general public and held 4-hour meetings using deliberative democracy methods to explain complex issues to attendees, giving them time to work through them and talk with colleagues about what might happen. Over the course of the year, the project engaged with 235 participants to discuss who would be prioritized if there were shortages of certain resources. Key messages included a community right to know and hope for a technological fix, such as sharing ventilators or using other technologies. But additionally, she noted that people were pragmatic and saw the need to be prepared against ad hoc approaches. They also did not want providers to be coming up with decisions as the needs arose. Finally, she said the participants held discussions around objective methods to combat biases, recognizing that biases can be ingrained within providers and systems, so community members wanted to ensure they were not embedded into any processes or decisions.

Will Stone, science reporter at National Public Radio, noted that most people had never heard of CSC before the pandemic emerged in early 2020. Once they did, early discussions focused on such extreme scenarios as having enough ventilators or beds for patients. The public opinion of CSC amounts to the assumption that people will be dying in the streets, he said. Headlines and language play a large role in this, and some evoke more fear than others. There is always a tension with how you describe the pandemic and current needs, he said, as you want to be concrete but also risk being reductive.

Reporting on the dire health care needs is difficult because it is not always clear to journalists when CSC is being activated, Stone noted. The media has to talk about this responsibly, but they are also very reliant on health officials to be clear about what is happening. There were many stories of full hospitals and shortages of workers, he explained, but it was never clear if that translated to CSC, so overall transparency to the press was lacking. Without that, it can be hard to get a nuanced portrait of what is truly happening in hospitals. People end up making CSC very black and white, stated Stone, even though it is not a light switch. Hick added that the field has struggled with triggers and understanding when the activations or details on shortages or changes in standards should be clearly communicated to the public.

REFLECTIONS

Mehta noted that these discussions highlight how complex CSC plans are and the immense amount of work that goes into avoiding these situations. He highlighted the need to reflect on how to engage with the community, how to think about equity, and how to deal with systemic imbalances within the health system. He also shared that he had not heard much of CSC until the pandemic emerged, but he realized as an intensivist there were many important allocation questions that would quickly emerge in his department if there were too many patients. Erin Serino, deputy chief of staff, Boston Emergency Medical Services, commented that she saw the trends in discussions as coordination and communication across systems and at state and regional levels. She pondered how to continue to drive that coordination and collaboration across states and at the national level. Shandiin Wood, health systems epidemiologist and tribal liaison, New Mexico Department of Health, agreed with coordination and collaboration being key, especially among disparate organizations across levels and geographies. He noted that to make these collaborations more effective, there is a clear need for better-integrated communication channels so that institutions are not geographically restricted when negotiating difficult questions about lack of resources.

Megan Jehn, associate professor, Arizona State University, added that as a nonclinician, most of her experience in CSC has been with community engagement. She reiterated the need to communicate in clear and consistent terms the differences in the needs of the various phases—conventional versus contingency versus crisis. In addition to the stress of living through a pandemic, she said, many communities carried the fear and stress of being on the receiving end of biases in these formalized processes and system protocols. She asked how to find best practices for gaining the public's trust. She noted there is also a need to maintain transparency and communicate to patients as they enter hospital systems so they are comfortable and trust that they are in a safe and just place. With all of the work that has happened in the last 18 months, Mehta concluded, this should reinvigorate stakeholders to push for these changes to be implemented in time for the next crisis. Given globalization and the movement of people across the world, there will certainly be another pandemic, but this is an opportunity to be better prepared.

5

Legal, Ethical, and Equity Considerations for Crisis Standards of Care

Critical legal, ethical, and equity aspects underlie the development and implementation of crisis standards of care (CSC) plans and processes. Providing legal and ethical support and guidance for providers can often alleviate much of the moral burden of making life-or-death decisions in a crisis or the uncertainty of delivering care in austere circumstances. In this chapter, speakers explore legal issues including liability protections and equity considerations related to the planning, activation, implementation, evaluation, and monitoring of CSC. Structured remarks from speakers are followed by a panel discussion and reflections on a way forward in these domains with the ongoing lessons gleaned from the COVID-19 pandemic.

LIABILITY PROTECTIONS: ISSUES AROUND MAKING TRIAGE DECISIONS

James Hodge, professor and director of the Center for Public Health Law and Policy at Arizona State University, began by restating IOM's original definition of CSC as a substantial change in usual health care operations and level of care because of a catastrophic disaster. CSC is implemented when sustained scarcities warrant real-time resource allocation to protect public health because the increased level of patient needs outweighs the available resources, such as intensive care unit (ICU) beds, personal protective equipment (PPE), medications, or health care workers. Hodge explained that there are many different legal topics involved in CSC, such as licensure, scope of practice, and documentation concerns, but a persistent and primary focus is protecting hospitals and clinicians against unwarranted risks of liability (Hodge et al., 2013). When navigating CSC and liability, there are many ethical and legal questions to consider, including:

- How do we allocate limited resources across systems?
- Who is responsible for life-or-death decisions?
- Who is liable if claims arise?

To answer these questions, clinicians and lawmakers must consider legal ways to allocate scarce resources. Hodge provided examples of legally prohibited allocation factors such as race, ethnicity, sex, and gender, and legally allowed allocation factors such as short-term survival, equitable clinical assessment scores, and specific resource limitations or suitability (Hodge et al., 2022). Health care workers, hospitals, triage committees, labs, emergency medical services, and public health officials all play a role in the allocation of scarce resources, he said, and all are subject to a web of liability risks, including civil, administrative, and criminal liability.

Hodge outlined two major approaches to avoiding CSC liability claims. First, health care institutions can simply follow the evolving standard of care by addressing what may be seen as a liability issue based on the crisis standard as implemented. Second, institutions could provide enhanced liability protections. There are multiple liability protections applicable to health care workers and volunteers, such as the Public Readiness and Emergency Preparedness Act, the Volunteer Protection Act, and the Good Samaritan Act. These laws protect providers from acts of negligence, but not gross negligence or intentional misconduct, he said. Hodge concluded with a reminder that there are limits to liability protections. Many liability protections can be claim specific or position specific, there can be jurisdictional variances, and some liability protections may last only for the duration of an emergency while others may provide comprehensive immunity.

Panel Discussion

Monica Peek, professor of medicine at the University of Chicago, moderated a panel discussing health care worker fears of liability, standards in place for triggering CSC, and the use of COVID-19 vaccination status in triage protocols. Robert Onders, administrator to the Alaska Native Medical Center, began by stating that Alaska currently does not have a public health emergency or CSC protocols on record. Valerie Gutmann Koch, director of law and ethics at the University of Chicago MacLean Center for Clinical Medical Ethics, added that during the pandemic, at least 37 states passed immunity protections for health care providers, but there were large state-by-state variations in levels of protection. Doug White, director for the Program on Ethics and Decision Making in Critical Illness at the University of Pittsburgh School of Medicine, discussed how many health care workers have concerns about lack of protections and fear the legal consequences that may arise when they must make difficult decisions of declining care to one patient to save another, even when such decisions explicitly follow state triage guidelines. He noted that while clinicians certainly need some protection when following legal triage guidelines, overly broad immunity can infringe on patient rights when a legitimate malpractice claim is raised.

Peek asked if standards for CSC are too high and whether clinicians operating under contingency standards of care may be more vulnerable to liability rather than those operating under crisis standards of care. Koch mentioned the vast amount of politicization that has surrounded CSC during the COVID-19 pandemic. There has been reluctance by some leaders to trigger CSC conditions or even acknowledge they exist, she said, something that has exacerbated inconsistencies in CSC between states. She pointed out that just because a state has signed off on implementing CSC, this does not mean it must be instituted at every hospital if conditions do not warrant it. Onders and White both agreed, and White added that there should be a prerequisite of load balancing before switching from contingency care to CSC. This would ensure that underfunded hospitals could receive resources from better equipped hospitals and potentially avoid needing to implement CSC, he explained.

Peek then asked about using COVID-19 vaccination status in triage protocols. White noted that, "while our quick emotional impulse is to consider vaccination status when triaging patients, we must consider the current political and social climate." He recounted the story of a recent experience with an unvaccinated patient dying from COVID-19. While this patient's family members were vaccinated, he said, the patient refused to be vaccinated because of reading information on Facebook stating there were "baby parts" in the vaccine. If patients were making truly informed decisions when deciding whether to get vaccinated against COVID-19, then it may be possible to consider vaccination status during triage, he said. However, considering vaccination status in a world with such toxic political discourse that allows people to make uninformed decisions may be an ethical gray area, whether these are caused by mistrust of the health system or poor health literacy.

A question from the audience asked about a *USA Today* article reporting 10,000 patients becoming infected with COVID-19 at a hospital while there for non-COVID-19 related appointments (Jewett, 2021). The article pointed to insufficient airborne precautions put in place by hospital administrators, placing patients infected with COVID-19 in rooms with patients who were negative for COVID-19, as well as a lack of infection control. A participant asked panelists if there are legal issues with the hospital's decisions in regard to CSC. Hodge stated that the hospital in the article may be liable if it were negligent in failing to implement basic precautions, and it is legally difficult to shield a hospital from liability in situations of gross negligence. Koch discussed how the standard of care is designed to be flexible and adapt to the current medical circumstances, including when resources are scarce or information about the pandemic is lacking. Onders provided an example of how his hospital shifted its standards of care during the COVID-19 pandemic by testing all admitted patients every 3 days and testing all patients prior to surgeries to ensure that patients sharing rooms were both negative for COVID-19.

Panelists also discussed the implications of the heterogeneity in CSC protocols at the local level across the country and the effects this has on both communities and physicians. Hodge stated that the antithesis of CSC is situations where multiple different hospitals in the same city are using entirely different CSC protocols when they are facing similar crisis conditions. This can create significant confusion at the local and regional level. Onders echoed this by sharing his experiences in Alaska, where hospitals with critical care capabilities varied in how they operated in contingency and CSC conditions, which created equity issues. White commented on hospitals' failures to achieve load balancing, highlighting that there is no reason for a hospital on one side of town to have depleted resources and become forced to implement CSC while a hospital on the other side of town has adequate resources they could share. This ultimately comes down to the inability to provide equitable care, since hospitals that often need to triage patients first are social safety net hospitals with little funding and staff. These hospitals are often located in more rural areas where disadvantaged communities, including people of color and poorer communities, are likely to seek care.

EQUITY AND THE ALLOCATION OF SCARCE RESOURCES

Govind Persad, assistant professor at Sturm College of Law, discussed the ethics behind the allocation of scarce resources and how to legally and ethically incorporate them into CSC. He stated that there is a broad spectrum of scarce resources. Scarce resources may involve critical care, such as lack of ventilators, health care workers, dialysis, or extracorporeal membrane oxygenation circuits, while scarce resources related to prevention may include monoclonal antibodies, antivirals, or vaccines. Ultimately, the objectives involved in equity and resource allocation are to (1) prevent harm, (2) mitigate health inequities, and (3) show equal concern for all recipients of care. He continued by discussing how predictive criteria can be used to categorize these three objectives by legal risk. Using predictive criteria such as health metrics like the sequential organ failure assessment (SOFA) score, occupational and caregiver status, and societal vulnerability metrics such as the Social Vulnerability Index (SVI) are ways to allocate resources that carry low legal risk. Triage protocols based on vaccination status, age, and specific health conditions carry a more moderate legal risk, he noted, while using criteria such as sex, gender, and race is legally prohibited, which Hodge noted earlier.

An alternative to predictive criteria, nonpredictive criteria, is another way to allocate scarce resources. Using a lottery or "first come, first served" approach is a way to randomly decide who receives care. However, Persad clarified, using nonpredictive criteria for resource allocation often fails to align or realize the objectives of preventing harm and mitigating health inequities as more disadvantaged groups die under the lottery approach (Tolchin et al., 2021). Finally, resource allocation can also be decided by combining criteria. Using priority point systems, where each criterion is assigned a point value, or categorized priority systems (e.g., 25 percent of monoclonal antibodies are prioritized for high SVI areas) are additional ways to ensure equity in resource allocation.

Persad also presented empirical findings to consider when aligning harm prevention and equity. When allocating ICU ventilators, taking an age-aware approach prevents more deaths and better mitigates racial inequities than using SOFA scores alone (Bhavani et al., 2021; Kesler et al., 2021; Raschke et al., 2021). As another example, for the COVID-19 vaccine allocation criteria, combining area deprivation measures with age better prevents harm and mitigates inequity than age alone (Wrigley-Field et al., 2021). COVID-19 has highlighted severe racial inequities in the U.S health care system as research shows racial minorities have died both of COVID-19 more often and earlier in life, Persad said, losing more years of life before age 65 than white victims (Bassett et al., 2020; Wortham et al., 2020). Generally speaking, he said, the public cares about saving lives during the COVID-19 pandemic, but opinions differ among older and younger generations regarding specific vaccination allocation criteria (Buckwalter and Peterson, 2020; Persad et al., 2021).

Persad concluded by suggesting areas of future research to improve equity during the allocation of scarce resources, such as ensuring fairness to non-COVID-19 patients. As the pandemic continues, non-COVID-19 patients have been denied care to make room for COVID-19 patients. He posed questions to be considered for future research to provide more insight into equitable resource allocation:

- Should hospitals reserve beds for non-COVID-19 patients?
- How does resource allocation change if a COVID-19 patient has refused the vaccine or other treatment such as monoclonal antibodies?
- How would the courts and the public view efforts to mitigate health inequity, such as using SVI scores, Medicaid recipient status, or race?

Discussion of Equity and Scarce Resource Allocation

During the subsequent panel discussion, Nneka Sederstrom, chief health equity officer of Hennepin Healthcare, offered thoughts on race within the context of allocating resources, saying that although it is an uncomfortable topic to discuss, it should not be shied away from when analyzing ways to reduce inequities. Using a color blind ideology does not work, she argued, as ignoring race does not create more equal care, it simply exacerbates inequities (Sederstrom and Wiggleton-Little, 2021). Virginia Brown, assistant professor in the Department of Population Health at Dell Medical School, discussed the mistrust that black and brown communities have in the health care system because their history with the health care system has been fraught with abuse and neglect, making it difficult to establish trust. She added that increasing community input when creating CSC and resource allocation standards will create a more transparent and trustworthy system by giving marginalized groups a seat at the table.

Sederstrom critiqued methods of resource allocation she thought of as being a proxy for race, such as the SVI or patient zip codes, and suggested using race itself as an allocation criteria would be more effective in reducing inequities. Persad noted that he viewed SVI as an attempt to reconcile intersecting disadvantages that often result from structural racism. He also pointed out that demographers have argued that using the census is a more effective way of tracking SVI and disadvantage indices than patient zip codes.

Thomas Sequist, chief patient experience and equity officer at Mass General Brigham, offered his thoughts on the lottery approach to resource allocation and his experience with disadvantaged indigenous populations. He stated that when systems such as lottery allocation are used, the assumption is made that the individuals entered into the lottery have equal access to health care. But not all patients in the lottery system have easy and reliable access to health resources and may find it difficult to access them even if they win the lottery. He discussed how indigenous populations are largely deprived of health care resources by being underfunded. While the U.S government spends, on average, approximately $10,000 per American per year on health care costs, it only spends around $4,500 per person per year for indigenous populations, he said. Sequist added that structural factors like systemic racism and poverty not only allowed COVID-19 to run rampant in indigenous communities, but such factors also play a role in traditional scoring systems such as SOFA scores for resource allocation.

He used the example of black communities having a three times higher incidence of kidney disease than the total population, a factor that would likely play a role when using a scoring system. Sequist noted that it is unfair for a scoring system to use the higher incidence of kidney disease against the black community, particularly when the reason for disease is because of hypertension, diet, and other factors that are a result of systemic racism. Systemic factors ultimately put black, brown, and poor communities at a disadvantage, he argued, both when trying to access health care resources and when a scoring system is used to allocate scarce resources.

Panelists were asked for their thoughts on how implicit bias and provider education on CSC perpetuates racism and ableism[1] in health care. Sequist stated that it is necessary to involve medical ethicists, or similar professionals with equal standing, along with the critical care physicians when providing input for creating CSC guidelines. An antiracism lens must be taken to all work being implemented as part of the COVID-19 pandemic response in order to proactively identify patients at risk for poor outcomes. These at-risk patients should then be contacted and provided with the resources and support needed to eliminate the possibility of poor outcomes from COVID-19, he said. Persad added that he would be interested in seeing more psychology research about how providers can minimize implicit bias.

When institutions fail to have clear and explicit CSC guidelines, providers can more easily activate their implicit bias when making treatment decisions. Persad explained that some of the most troubling stories of bias were not situations where there was a biased standard of care, but where there was no standard of care, leaving clinicians to make choices that appeared to be based on race. Sederstrom concluded by stating that for any substantive change to occur, building empathy is needed. Without empathy, she said, biases and cultural norms can take hold. Including empathy in CSC guidelines and scarce resource allocation will allow clinicians to make informed, equitable decisions that are in the best interest of patients.

REFLECTIONS

Suzet McKinney, principal and director of Life Sciences; Jennifer Piatt, deputy director of the Network for Public Health Law–Western Region Office; and Cynda Rushton, professor and chair of Johns Hopkins School of Nursing, offered their thoughts on the legal and ethical discussions. McKinney shared her experience in Chicago where initially there was much hesitancy towards CSC planning because it was difficult to fathom a scenario where it would ever need to be implemented. The allocation of scarce resources has always been the elephant in the room when thinking about CSC, she noted, but COVID-19 has highlighted the need for robust planning and collaboration across all levels of government. Piatt added that lack of CSC planning leads to situations where providers are making

---

[1] Ableism is defined as the discrimination or prejudice against individuals with disabilities.

ad hoc, nonuniform decisions that affect patients differently based on their location.

Rushton said that physicians have not been adequately prepared for the moral residue that comes with making CSC decisions. The COVID-19 pandemic has forced clinicians to make difficult decisions about the allocation of scarce resources, and it is essential that proper triage guidelines are in place and health care workers receive support when faced with making such tough decisions. Rushton also suggested considering if the threshold for implementing CSC is too high. She echoed Sederstrom's previous comments about empathy. Because COVID-19 has depleted the workforce and drained health care workers of the ability to empathize, reevaluating the appropriate time to trigger CSC conditions and instituting them earlier may better preserve resources in all forms, including health care workers.

Piatt and Rushton offered their perspectives on the true reason providers and institutions are worried about liability: fear. Emergency circumstances highlight how important liability protections are when a crisis warrants all hands on deck. The COVID-19 pandemic has caused a shortage in health care workers and created a circumstance where any and all help from clinicians is needed. Without liability protections, some health care workers may be hesitant to step up in times of crisis owing to fear of legal repercussions. Liability protections will increase the willingness of providers to step up during an emergency, Piatt explained. However, she questioned if such protections will truly increase the reliance and implementation of CSC when the opportunity arises.

Rushton concluded by stating that the health care system has been relationally depleted by the COVID-19 pandemic. The key to getting through these difficult times is not to think our way through, she said, but to feel our way through and listen to one another wholeheartedly. Clinicians need a heavy dose of humility when it comes to CSC planning and allocation of scarce resources. By not letting go of professional expertise, not listening, and not engaging with the communities we aim to serve, their health and wellness may be jeopardized, Rushton concluded.

Eric Toner, senior scholar and scientist for the Center for Health Security at Johns Hopkins University, concluded by saying we all have the duty to plan and prepare. Many liability issues stem from the fact that institutions fail to do the work involved to prepare for CSC conditions. Many hospitals have also failed to achieve load balancing, a practice that when done correctly could save many lives. Evaluating when CSC situations are implemented is just as important as how they are implemented, he continued. CSC conditions should be triggered when institutions recognize that their resources have become limited, rather than when their state government recognizes it. When considering how to allocate scarce resources, health care workers must be included in those conversations and recognized as a critical resource that must be used in the best way to avoid burnout. To establish more trust and create more equity, Toner emphasized community engagement and seeking community opinions on CSC planning rather than waiting for the community's reaction to plans that have already been created. Communities are willing and able to have the tough discussions, he said, and they want to contribute.

6

Looking Forward

More than any other event since the conception and emergence of CSC plans in 2009, the COVID-19 pandemic has tested how well these plans work. Throughout this experience, lessons have been learned that can inform future planning and give jurisdictions who are just now learning about this framework options to leap past much of the experiential learning that had to take place over the past 10 years. In this chapter, speakers highlight the experiences of CSC at the federal level and the potential roles for the federal government going forward. A subsequent panel discussion synthesizes the challenges and opportunities across key areas of CSC, as previously discussed throughout this workshop series: staffing; planning and implementation; and legal, ethical, and equity considerations. The chapter concludes with a reflection on the opportunities for CSC as the COVID-19 pandemic continues and as leaders and responders continue to consider the risk of the emergence of new pathogens.

KEYNOTE PRESENTATIONS

David Christian Hassell, senior science advisor, deputy assistant secretary for preparedness and response, Office of the Assistant Secretary for Preparedness and Response (ASPR) within HHS, recounted his initial encounter with the 2009 CSC set when he arrived at the ASPR office in 2019. However, once COVID-19 emerged, he said, ASPR realized that CSC needed another look given that it would likely play a role as the pandemic unfolded. From the beginning, ASPR has been very concerned about the effect on frontline health workers and has tried to understand the various needs of different settings. Essentially, ASPR's goal is to understand how to help clinicians provide the highest benefit to patients, Hassell said.

Richard Hunt, senior medical advisor, National Health Care Preparedness Programs, ASPR, shared some observations after listening to many clinicians throughout the pandemic. "We really didn't have a lot of experience implementing CSC before," he said, "but now we have learned quite a bit." While listening to frontline workers and the general public about their thoughts related to CSC is important, Hunt said, it needs to be paired with the years of work spent on planning and learn from those who have clinical bedside experience with CSC. He added that the implementation of CSC across the country, with or without planning and standards, outlined the challenges that come with CSC. At its core, CSC happens between patients and their health care team. Some providers had little to no awareness of CSC prior to having to make life-or-death decisions for their patients. Moral injury, compassion fatigue, and attacks on clinicians are becoming more prevalent, said Hunt. Many providers are walking away from medicine. He shared an example in Montana where in some regions, 9-1-1 calls via EMS are met with no response (Montana DPHHS et al., 2021).

CSC addresses the times when there are scarce resources available, especially given the health care workforce shortage—which will likely last for years. Hunt pointed out that the health care delivery system in the United States has become diminished in its capability and capacity. He asked how the nation could best address this profound challenge, and how it could support clinicians to deliver the best care possible when they do have to implement CSC without indicators and standards. If there is no room in curriculums and continued learning for CSC, Hunt asked, then how can the federal government best support clinicians either in real-time when they are faced with difficult decisions, or after they have made them and are left with profound mental anguish? Acknowledging the fatigue that many providers feel and how that affects work on CSC, Hunt stated that based on the experience throughout the pandemic, iterative thinking will not work. He concluded that there is a need to be bold and open minded in thinking about changes, and this kind of an opportunity may only come once in a century.

Roles for the Federal Government

Hassell said the more that federal agencies can provide all the CSC tools in advance for clinicians and policy makers at the state and local levels, the better. There is a great deal of focus on the technical and scientific aspects, he explained, but there is also a need to talk about nontechnical aspects, including the administration of programs and education by politicians and bureaucrats. Federal agencies have a role, but they cannot do it alone, and they need to partner with other organizations to be successful. Hunt added that, being involved in some way with the development of CSC over the years, he has learned that denial is a powerful tool. Nobody wants to do this, he said. Whether it is a clinician at the bedside, hospital leadership, or the general public, no one wants to have these conversations. When working with various jurisdictions and clinicians, the whole idea is "out of sight, out of mind," he explained. But providing tools and finding areas where the people can engage with state and local officials has more receptivity now compared to before the pandemic. He cautioned not to underestimate how difficult this process is. He also agreed with Hassell that involvement from federal agencies is not a magic bullet solution. Grassroots approaches and clinicians familiar with ethical concepts who embrace the process are critical.

The federal government has been accomplishing a great deal in this area, but it is frustrating that many clinicians have never heard of CSC, said Eric Toner, senior scholar, Center for Health Security, Johns Hopkins University. He wondered what else could be done to address this and get the attention of those who need to hear this. Hunt replied that using whatever levers are available to make this into clinician education training would be valuable. There is extraordinary variability in the awareness of clinicians about CSC, and many just do the "best they can" and do not connect their decisions at all with the concepts and established frameworks of CSC. Hassell added that more input is needed. ASPR has been reaching out to broad groups of stakeholders, but Hassel said he is interested to know what others think the federal government and national academies can do to help support this effort. Toner finished by saying we should think of ways to not only revise guidance but also to better disseminate and foster its adoption.

REFLECTIONS ON CHALLENGES AND OPPORTUNITIES

This section brings together the topics discussed throughout the workshop series. Speakers summarized the targeted discussions and offered either future questions to consider or key lessons to inform planning across the areas of staffing; planning and implementation; and legal, ethical, and equity issues.

Staffing Considerations

Tener Goodwin Veenema, professor of nursing, Johns Hopkins Center for Health Security, reviewed some of the goals of their discussion, including articulating the opportunities highlighted in Chapter 3 to improve the CSC framework and guidance for planning, activation, implementation, evaluation, and monitoring. She acknowledged the challenges ahead when thinking about not only future staffing needs but also considering the long-term effect on the health care workforce.

First, Veenema recounted some statements and findings discussed in Chapter 3. The moral injury and staff attrition in health care have been profound, she said, with 30 percent considering leaving their profession. She also noted that 60 percent reported experiencing negative effects on their mental health as a result of their work throughout the pandemic. She mentioned the confusion over the difference between moving from contingency mode to crisis mode, and the allocation of scarce resources decisions left to providers at the bedside. She also highlighted the travel nursing industry, which has contributed to many staffing challenges for hospitals and health care centers.

Challenges include obstacles to mobilizing staff, realizing institutions were not very good at predicting staffing needs, and the need for better cross-sector collaboration across the health care disciplines. There was also a loss of team cohesion, she noted, which has a negative effect on efficiency and trust during difficult patient care situations. This is especially amplified when there are new staff or rotating providers who are not familiar with institutional policies and protocols. For a future framework of CSC staffing needs, she offered several ideas, issues, and strategies:

- Use technology more effectively to resolve or alleviate staffing burden issues (allow nursing care delivery to include telenursing and the e-ICU),
- Better data collection,
- Collected data needs to be shared with relevant parties to be more useful,
- Improve collaboration and communication with entities crossing state borders (e.g., load balancing, EMS, e-ICUs), and
- Create a built-in ethical framework for staffing during CSC implementation.

Veenema reiterated some of the immediate, short-term, and long-term strategies that some large integrated health care centers are using (see Figure 3-3). She also noted the inflection point of two concurrent crises happening in November 2021—the Delta variant and its resulting surge of unvaccinated patients coupled with the burnout crisis of the health care workforce. Physicians are closing practices, there has been an increase in suicides and suicidal ideations in health care professionals, and nurses are leaving the workforce, she explained. She asked how best to correct these and build in respite care to give the workforce time to take a breath and build much-needed resilience. She also wondered what could be done to the workforce pipeline to mitigate future shortages.

Gregg Meyers, president of the Community Division and executive vice president of value-based care at Mass General Brigham, addressed the ongoing challenge of trying to preserve the health care workforce and finding the balance between resilience and workforce stressors. Trying to attend to the hierarchy of needs among colleagues includes ensuring our workforce is sufficiently prepared for these events and feels supported, Meyers added. Workers also need to feel recognized and honored for the work they do. He outlined several foundational elements for the future, based on creating a safe and nurturing workplace setting (see Box 3-1).

Meyers also highlighted some of the key administrative considerations in staffing, including the perverse payment structures that finance the nursing and technical workforce, and he wondered how to invest in nursing differently. As many learned, providing childcare turns out to be absolutely essential to responding to a long-term event and keeping people in the workforce. While this previously seemed outside the purview of health care, it is now front and center.

He also noted the suggestion that there should be a federal overarching coordinating body for CSC. He offered that it could be housed within ASPR and could have the scope of authority to mobilize the resources necessary to respond. This body could also provide a pulse check, he said, and be able to assess staffing numbers nationally and provide situational awareness on what is happening around the country. Finally, Meyers said being able to provide virtual care and harness technology in the e-ICU has been such a jump forward. The ability to virtually move staff through time and space is something that has never been done.

Future Changes to Improve Workforce Needs

Mike Wargo, vice president and chief, Enterprise Preparedness and Emergency Operations, HCA Healthcare, highlighted the notion of the cross-sector alliance, but said we need a stronger bond between health care and public health leaders. He suggested reevaluating the health care incident management system and educating health care leaders more on this unified model and how everyday surges are typically managed. He also called for embracing the future workforce—looking to academia and educating future nurses and emergency managers on CSC. He argued that the workforce should be given the opportunity to understand what to expect in hopes of changing the culture, said Wargo. As Meyers mentioned, many current workers are nearing retirement, and the Medical Reserve Corps (MRC), the national network of medical volunteers, should acknowledge that and prepare itself as best as possible. Wargo noted that the MRC had been left to stagnate, but when COVID-19 suddenly emerged, the health care system needed to rely on it. He suggested encouraging those around the country who are retiring now or in the short term to join the MRC unit closest to them.

Finally, he advocated for a unified mission and vision. Wargo concluded that if a common vision of what crisis looks like was shared, then the community would be able to come together, which would lead to better outcomes. Asha Devereaux, senior medical officer, Sharp Coronado Hospital, also added that outpatient providers and their teams are typically not included in CSC planning. As seen throughout the COVID-19 pandemic, CSC happened in the outpatient world as well. "Whether patients selected to do hospice at home and avoid crowded hospital settings, they will need our support," she concluded.

Planning and Implementation

Anuj Mehta, assistant professor of medicine, Denver Health and Hospital Authority, reflected on some of the challenges his team identified around planning and implementation, saying when thinking about moving from plans to reality, they considered implementation case studies, workforce preparation challenges, decision-making challenges, and public and stakeholder perceptions. There has been a lot of debate about how to triage patients for ventilators, he said, or guiding decisions about things that cannot be anticipated in a crisis that may evolve over time. The workshop on planning and implementation highlighted that situational awareness should drive decision making relating to CSC development and planning, as well as activation, implementation, evaluation, and monitoring.

Health care is not the best at real-time assessment, he noted, as has been discussed previously, but many things emerged across speakers and conversations that can and should inform future work. He listed key lessons concerning community engagement, coordination and collaboration, and the workforce (Box 6-1).

Mehta noted that CSC should not be just triage. Supporting mental health in addition to basic human resources staffing is critical (see Figure 6-1). CSC is a deviation from the standard of care where care to patients is degraded to what would be considered acceptable. He said the line between contingency and crisis is often blurred and that this is where the discomfort arises being a physician. He also suggested considering reducing nonurgent procedures, load balancing, or altering standard therapy—as all of these things may happen before a formal triage protocol for CSC is implemented. This continuum presents a risk to the moral and ethical duties that clinicians have, as well as adding to licensure and liability concerns. He echoed past comments on the importance of presenting this type of event as a continuum related to an ongoing crisis rather than a dichotomous switch that turns on and off.

> **BOX 6-1**
> **Key Lessons for CSC Planning and Implementation**
>
> **Community Engagement**
>
> - Engage with community members early and often to build trust.
> - Ensure inclusive and diverse representation from the community.
> - Structurally marginalized communities are fearful of discrimination and implicit bias.
> - Messaging around CSC is complex and needs to maintain transparency while not inducing panic.
>
> **Coordination and Collaboration**
>
> - There are challenges associated with staffing and tracking equipment and supplies across hospitals and health care systems.
> - Maintaining situational awareness, resource sharing, and load balancing have been challenging.
> - Individual facility activations versus regional activations are variable and difficult to standardize.
> - There may be consistent ethical principles on paper, but the actual implementation of them may vary across systems.
>
> **Workforce**
>
> - Staffing has evolved as a key driver of resource scarcity over the course of the pandemic.
> - Clinicians are worried about threats to their individual decision making, autonomy, and moral and ethical duty to the patient.
> - There needs to be more transparency and communication with the workforce about CSC planning.
> - Management and hospital administrations should support the workforce throughout the activation, implementation, and duration of CSC.
>
> SOURCE: Anuj Mehta presentation, November 22, 2021.

The scarcity goes beyond discrete devices like ventilators, Mehta continued. Throughout the pandemic, health care systems have experienced shortages of various staff types and shortages of medications, oxygen, or dialysis machines. There are also patients that may be downgraded to a lower level of care than they typically would receive. Now health care is facing shortages across the entire system, he noted, and not just ventilators. Thinking beyond the basic allocation of scarce resources related to types of devices or supplies, he presented a broad framework for CSC, and posited

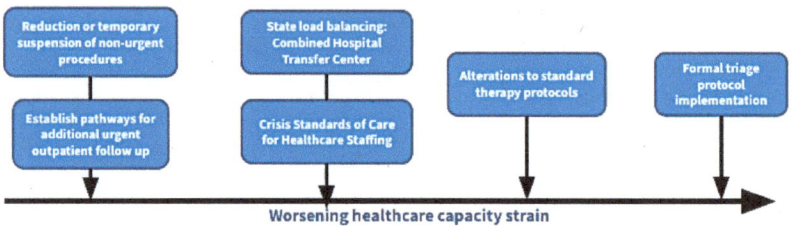

Crisis Continuum

FIGURE 6-1 Worsening health care capacity strain throughout the crisis continuum.
SOURCE: Anuj Mehta presentation, November 22, 2021.

the following questions to guide a more global framework when deciding how best to allocate scarce resources:

- How likely is a patient to survive without the resource being considered?
- How likely is a patient to not need readmission or reevaluation without the resource considered?
- How likely is a patient to survive even if they do receive the resource being considered?
- Does the patient have realistic access to an alternate care pathway if they are triaged to it (e.g., outpatient care including follow-up, equipment, supplies, and medications)?

While CSC is a continuum, Mehta said, it also involves a host of decision-making points that we may think about today but cannot anticipate what they will be tomorrow. He called for a framework to guide practice both ethically and practically. He concluded that the one key lesson learned is that there will be another crisis, so this is an opportunity to create systems that can perform better next time.

Discussion

Toner asked how the benefits of moving resources from one group to another can be assessed. For example, moving staff members around or cancelling elective procedures to take care of COVID-19 patients has been done, but no one has talked about whether the real effect—benefit or harm—is known. Mehta agreed this is an important question and comes with other key related questions. How do you evaluate this in real time? Are we achieving the benefit we want? Are we identifying patients most likely to survive? Patients need to be tracked during triage, he said, not just left to wait until the crisis is over. There also needs to be real-time equity evaluations.

Inequities built into the health care system have been exacerbated in this pandemic, Mehta said. Lots of scoring systems have inequities too, he noted, so providers and hospital leaders need to evaluate inequity in all situations where care is being delivered. Those living in rural areas or who have low insurance coverage may be presenting to a hospital much later in their illness progression, and thus have more severe disease because they do not have accessible services. What should we be thinking about regarding how the shifting of resources that occurred affected other patients, both short term and long term, to inform decisions for the next crisis. Where can the health care system actually expand? What are the downstream consequences when the system shrinks back? There is a need to further research these questions to inform the planning for the next crisis, he concluded.

Toner asked who should be involved in making these critical triage decisions. Mehta responded that there are established large-scale frameworks and scores that may be adopted at a state level, but there is a need to consider key stakeholders when doing that. At the ground level in the hospital, he argued for the need to remove this responsibility from the health care providers at the bedside, who are naturally invested in getting their patients the best possible outcome. Having a more objective group of people who have the right expertise and who are also a bit removed from direct care, and who are able to make these decisions, is paramount.

Shandiin Wood, health systems epidemiologist and tribal liaison, New Mexico Department of Health, said that one thing to learn from this experience is the importance of adherence to the plan in a consistent format across different sites, hospitals, and regions within the state. If there is a consistent implementation of a framework adoption, he said, then you have the benefit of looking at intermediate outcomes and fidelity of the adopted plan, which can then provide insight into the long-term effects. This is better than a haphazard adoption of frameworks at different hospitals across the same region, which has happened in many places. He emphasized the need to standardize health and survival outcomes in a given area for people who have gone through that framework.

Legal, Ethical, and Equity Considerations

Jennifer Piatt, deputy director, Network for Public Health Law–Western Region Office, reviewed the webinar discussion dedicated to legal challenges and opportunities pertaining to liability protections in CSC, as well as the incorporation of ethical and equity considerations in the allocation of scarce resources. Piatt said there are two approaches during CSC implementation. The first involves following the standard of care and evolving with changing circumstances, so the standard of care shifts as needed. But there are distinct concerns in this pathway, she said. It becomes extremely difficult to assess retroactively where a particular standard shifted in a particular location at a particular time. There are lots of different interpretations on that standard; without uniformity, the state, local, and hospital plans all differ.

The second pathway provides enhanced liability protections and may provide more comfort for providers who know that they are supported. But questions for this pathway include duration of the protections and scope of immunity provided. Protections may only last during an emergency declaration, Piatt explained, and may only apply to specific persons or behavior. For example, she reviewed two legal sources for liability protection at the federal level. The CARES Act provides express liability protections for interstate volunteer health care workers, in contrast with the PREP Act, which applies to all covered health care workers against claims of loss in response to a public health emergency. Additional protections can differ at the state level across jurisdictions, resulting in a confusing patchwork of protections at different times for different people or entities.

The second area Piatt highlighted is nondiscrimination in CSC and making difficult decisions lawfully during emergencies. The HHS Office of Civil Rights set up the three categories of red, yellow, and green light scenarios included in triage plans to help guide decisions. She explained that clearly impermissible bases are legally prohibited allocations, which involve categorical exclusions based on protected criteria. She added that the list should be considered as "evolving" as additional evidence arises to illustrate additional disparate effects of other possible allocations bases. CSC plans need to go beyond simply identifying express discrimination and address issues that perpetuate systemic inequities, like SOFA scoring. Planning must be deliberate in addressing disparities, she said.

Monica Peek, professor of medicine, University of Chicago, transitioned to thinking about explicitly ethical issues. The large question with CSC, she said, is can we align multiple different ethical goals? In other words, can we try to prevent harm such as death or illness, as well as loss of caregivers? Can people be treated with equal concern? Can health disparities be mitigated? For those who have been facing structural disadvantages, she asked, how do we as a society take into consideration that their lives have been harmed by policies and procedures that have put them at a disadvantage over time? These people come into health systems with an extra burden of "dis-health" and disease, she noted.

Some research is showing promise for the alignment of these goals. For example, within the ICU, studies have shown that age-aware approaches prevent more deaths and better mitigate racial inequity than SOFA alone

(Raschke et al., 2021). When we think about the distribution of COVID-19 vaccines, Peek said, combining age and SVI is better at preventing harm and mitigating inequity than age alone (Wrigley-Field et al., 2021). She noted the increasing ways being discovered to use these principles in a synergistic fashion to achieve more goals. There are several challenges with mitigation of health disparities. Some categories are not legally allowed to be considered, such as those in the red list, as Piatt had previously noted, but others, while sometimes controversial, can be considered—such as age, vaccination status, SVI, and health metrics.

The previous workshop dedicated to this topic (detailed in Chapter 5) included much discussion around race, but the racial health disparities were amplified and seen the most in news headlines during the COVID-19 pandemic. Peek asked what are the best ways to address those disparities most effectively and comprehensively, and whether this should be done by thinking about individual race, group-level race (including structural disadvantage), or racism. She pondered whether it could be achieved by working exclusively within current legal constraints, or by thinking about a longer historical narrative where there is an understanding that laws were not always just and it has been part of our country's history to push back against laws that may not be fair—especially for racial and ethnic minorities. Peek suggested the most justice might be found by pushing back against laws and fully capturing racial equity in decision systems for CSC. Solely looking at some of the mechanisms through which structural racism occurs, she said, will make it difficult to develop ways to mitigate health disparities most effectively.

When thinking about scarce resource allocation in the ICU, the resources that come to mind most often are things like ventilators, but as others have mentioned, leaders should be expanding their own mindsets to also think about people, monoclonal antibodies, and other critical resources that may become scarce. She commented that one topic that has been prevalent throughout the webinar series has been the hospital transfer systems and their role in mitigating inequities. That is the most important next frontier in trying to mitigate health inequities—thinking about load balancing at the community level, Peek noted. It is important to consider that small hospitals, often serving communities of color, are most often overrun while tertiary care systems, which primarily serve white communities, have more resources and capacity. She concluded that keeping this in mind when facilitating load balancing can promote equity.

Ethical Reactions to the Pandemic

Matt Wynia, director, Center for Bioethics and Humanities, University of Colorado, said many of the challenges experienced in the pandemic were expected, but we did not know the extent to which they were going to come into play. For example, the critical importance of load balancing to avoid going into CSC emerged in several locations as a potential preventive measure. Early in the pandemic in New York City, he said, it was more understandable that some hospitals were forced into contingency modes while others nearby had empty beds, as everyone was still figuring things out. But he referred to a story in Texas where just a few months ago a young man died of a curable illness because a hospital bed could not be found. That is completely inexcusable at this point in the pandemic, he argued.

Wynia also commented on the reticence health care institutions had about entering CSC and no longer being able to offer standard services to their population, saying he and his colleagues did expect some of that hesitation. But they did not realize the degree to which hospitals and states would wait and avoid authorizing and activating CSC. By the time organizations actually admit they are at that point, he said, they've been there for weeks, if not months. He noted that Colorado had declared CSC for certain things, but many institutions and providers are doing things right now that are quite risky, and doing them without protections.

Finally, he pointed out the irony of CSC documents clearly stating up front that such factors as race, age, and socioeconomic status are not used in allocations and algorithms, but it has become clear during the pandemic that sometimes those do have to be used. For example, early on when authorities were talking about ventilator allocation in several places, the focus was very much on who would die even if they got a ventilator. But thinking about discharge, he said, we now need to consider these types of factors because you cannot ethically discharge someone without insurance coverage or social supports even though they clinically might be the best case to get discharged. Additionally, when age was used for vaccine allocation and distribution there was very little pushback, and elderly people were happy to be first in line. But for other things, like ICU allocation, people were not happy to see age being used as a reason not to receive an ICU bed. So even within our own field, Wynia concluded, there are tensions about how best to use these kinds of criteria.

LOOKING TO THE FUTURE

Suzet McKinney, principal and director of Life Sciences at Sterling Bay, outlined where we can learn and inform planning. Previously, there were a few examples where there were opportunities to gain experience with CSC, such as the Ebola outbreak and certain hurricanes. But at this point, she explained, there has been enough opportunity to do a reevaluation of CSC to ensure all the necessary components of the framework are included and have been informed through our response to COVID-19. There is also enough evidence and experience at this point to provide recommendations on how to implement the framework. This is a great opportunity to advise others on how to use the framework and how to implement it in the most effective way while also ensuring that health care workers are well trained on indicators and triggers.

Certainly, COVID-19 took us by surprise, McKinney continued, but there were moments throughout the response, especially early on, when we could have anticipated much sooner some of those things that were going to affect our health care systems and ability to implement public health strategies. She amplified Veenema's previous comments on nurses being a scarce resource and taking that into account more seriously in planning efforts. Another aspect that has been discussed for some time is the need for a toolkit or framework for elected officials. Clearly the scope and size of COVID-19 had officials much more involved than previous emergency responses, McKinney said, but there is now a great impetus for an elected official toolkit at this point.

There is an opportunity to develop a communications framework that integrates messaging at all levels of government so we are providing the most up-to-date and succinct information to the American public, she noted. She also supported the idea of creating a federal coordinating body, which could assist in developing this government communications framework but also could assist in implementing the framework should it become necessary. Finally, she was reminded of the pandemic influenza exercises at the national level that CDC used to conduct with specific jurisdictions to assist them in exercising their plans and measuring effectiveness. There are opportunities at this point to conduct multilevel government and jurisdictional exercises specifically around CSC plans to measure progress at the state and local levels and identify areas for improvement, she concluded.

Wynia highlighted some of the things that he used to worry about before the pandemic and that he now worries about differently. In the aftermath of earlier outbreaks such as SARS in 2003 and Ebola in 2015, he was concerned that politicians would overreact to infectious disease outbreaks and overuse public health police powers to stoke panic or needlessly overreach and be counterproductive. But now he worries about that differently, he explained. Politicians are not doing what they need to be doing right now during the COVID-19 pandemic. So, the role of the public health and medical enterprise in serving as a counterweight to political considerations is different than he anticipated it to be, he said. He stated he originally thought politicians would have to be held back, but instead some had to be pushed forward.

Secondly, he noted the large amount of work done on the "duty to treat" for health professionals and getting them to show up in the face of risk. Wynia stated that early in the pandemic that was not a problem, as collegiality and volunteerism were at high levels. People did not even need legal protections—they showed up for dangerous and difficult work even when about to retire, he added. But now, Wynia explained, 18 months in, people are burning out and retiring. People can only be stretched so far until they break, he said. So, this conversation for him has changed to how do professionals in the field support frontline workers to maintain their resilience. He is also thinking more about how to encourage members of the public to ask themselves what are *their* duties as citizens? He believes it possible to have a national consensus on the ethical framework for CSC, as certain questions do get at core actions where there would be wide consensus. But there are numerous implementation challenges that would prove difficult.

Dan Hanfling, vice president, technical staff, In-Q-Tel, offered a few reflections from his experience with CSC over the past decade. He stated that never in a million years did he think that in the greatest health crisis of our time that he would see an erosion of trust in health care workers and public health authorities. He also never anticipated the level of political dysfunction that hampered the country's ability to put in place what was required for a robust response. With that as context, Hanfling offered a few things about the framework and then suggested some steps to consider going forward, noting the framework was still relevant and aligned with CSC goals and parameters. He recognized that there is a duty to plan and prepare, as well as a duty to steward resources.

Past stakeholders who have worked on these issues over the years all knew that it was always a matter of when, not if, Hanfling said; they knew it was going to happen. He commented on the age of epidemics happening now, with SARS-CoV-2 being the third coronavirus outbreak in 17 years. There are going to be more crises like these, he cautioned. He elaborated on Wynia's previous point, about engagement at all levels, and thinking about it more ethically, alongside a concept of reciprocity. Looking back on the ethical framework we focused mostly on accountability, Hanfling explained, motivated by the searing testimonials in the aftermath of Hurricane Katrina. There were strong feelings that the government should be accountable to its people at that time, but now it has become clear that people should also be accountable to their communities.

The lack of preparedness clearly relates to liability, he continued. Situational awareness became a critical element early in the process. Load balancing became the operative phrase to get the patients to the right place at the right time with the right resources, but without a national data infrastructure, this was a very difficult task. He called for prioritizing the development of something like that, as technology can be a force multiplier. There is an opportunity to deliver on capabilities like remote patient monitoring, telemedicine, and artificial intelligence, he said, and smarter ways to deliver care, where just a few years ago these types of assets were only seen in the movies.

As a few final points, Hanfling shared that currently, such quantitative measures as SOFA scoring are unfulfilling, and there is a need to move away from that and identify better and more equitable measures. It also is important to recognize the need for clarity on indicators and triggers and being able to know when a crisis should be declared in terms of altering standards of care. Right now, this happens at the bedside, Hanfling said, but it is important to consider how to shift that decision to the left chronologically, and be able to prevent haphazard decisions from being made on an individual basis. Instead, through good situational awareness, hospital leaders should be able to declare a change of standards across the board prior to things falling apart. In summary, he offered four suggestions CSC work could focus on:

1. There should be better and broader coordination and understanding between the bedside and board room. This is an "all of health care entity" requirement, and that divide needs to be bridged.
2. Increase buy-in from the political sector. Politicians need to understand what is happening and be active participants in the process.
3. Expand provider engagement, which has been an area of underinvestment previously but can be very valuable.
4. Effectively address health equity issues. Whether it is COVID-19, masks, or structural racism, it is important as a nation to do better.

References

Bassett, M. T., J. T. Chen, and N. Krieger. 2020. Variation in racial/ethnic disparities in COVID-19 mortality by age in the United States: A cross-sectional study. *PLOS Medicine* 17(10):e1003402.

Bhavani, S. V., Y. Luo, W. D. Miller, L. N. Sanchez-Pinto, X. Han, C. Mao, B. Sandikçi, M. E. Peek, C. M. Coopersmith, K. N. Michelson, and W. F. Parker. 2021. Simulation of ventilator allocation in critically ill patients with COVID-19. *American Journal of Respiratory Critical Care Medicine* 204(10):1224-1227.

Buckwalter, W., and A. Peterson. 2020. Public attitudes toward allocating scarce resources in the COVID-19 pandemic. *PLOS ONE* 15(11):e0240651.

Ehmann, M. R., E. Zink, A. Levin, J. Suarez, H. Belcher, E. Daugherty Biddison, D. Doberman, K. D'Souza, D. Fine, B. Garibaldi, E. Gehrie, S. Golden, A. Gurses, P. Hill, M. Hughes, J. Kahn, C. Koch, J. Marx, B. Meisenberg, J. Natterman, C. Rushton, A. Sapirstein, S. Selinger, R.S. Stephens, E. Toner, Y. Unguru, M. van Stone, A. Kachalia. 2021. Operational recommendations for scarce resource allocation in a public health crisis. *Chest* 159(3):1076-1083. https://doi.org/10.1016/j.chest.2020.09.246.

Garrett, A. L. 2020. Adapting a federal disaster medical assistance team to operate during a pandemic. *Disaster Medicine and Public Health Preparedness* 23:1-3. https://doi.org/10.1017/dmp.2020.405.

Hodge, J. G., D. Hanfling, and T. Powell. 2013. Practical, ethical, and legal challenges underlying crisis standards of care. *Journal of Law, Medicine, and Ethics* 41(S1):50-55.

Hodge, J. G , J. L. Piatt, and R. Freed. 2022. Navigating legalities in crisis standards of care. *Maryland Journal of Health Care Law and Policy* (forthcoming). https://ssrn.com/abstract=4014599 (accessed March 26, 2022).

HHS (U.S. Department of Health and Human Services). 2009. *Federal assessment finds progress, gaps in state plans for pandemic influenza.* http://wayback.archive-it.org/3926/20131018161737/http://www.hhs.gov/news/press/2009pres/01/20090115i.html (accessed January 26, 2022).

HHS. 2021. *OCR provides technical assistance to ensure crisis standards of care protect against age and disability discrimination.* https://www.hhs.gov/about/news/2021/01/14/ocr-provides-technical-assistance-ensure-crisis-standards-of-care-protect-against-age-disability-discrimination.html (accessed January 26, 2022).

IOM (Institute of Medicine). 2009. *Guidance for establishing crisis standards of care for use in disaster situations.* Washington, DC: National Academies Press.

IOM. 2012. *Crisis standards of care: A systems framework for catastrophic disaster response, Volume 1: Introduction and CSC framework.* Washington, DC: The National Academies Press. https://doi.org/10.17226/13351 (accessed March 26, 2022).

Jewett, C. 2021. Patients went into the hospital for care. After testing positive there for COVID-19, some never came out. *USA Today.* https://www.usatoday.com/story/news/nation/2021/11/04/patients-admitted-hospitals-unrelated-ailment-left-covid/6263682001 (accessed January 26, 2022).

Kesler, S. M., J. T. Wu, K. R. Kalland, L. G. Peter, J. K. Wothe, J. K. Needle, Q. Wang, and C. R. Weinert. 2021. Operationalizing ethical guidance for ventilator allocation in Minnesota: Saving the most lives or exacerbating health disparities? *Critical Care Explorations* 3(6):e0455.

Kirzinger, A., A. Kearney, L. Hamel, and M. Brodie. 2021. *KFF/The Washington Post Frontline Health Care Workers Survey.* Washington, DC: Kaiser Family Foundation/Washington Post.

Montana DPHHS, Montana Hospital Association, and the Montana Healthcare Foundation. 2021. *Emergency medical services in Montana: Crisis on the horizon.* https://dphhs.mt.gov/assets/publichealth/EMSTS/EMS/EMSSurveyReport.pdf (accessed January 26, 2022).

Parker, W. F., G. Persad, and M. E. Peek. 2021. Four recommendations to efficiently and equitably accelerate the COVID-19 vaccine rollout. *Health Affairs Blog.* https://www.healthaffairs.org/do/10.1377/forefront.20210204.166874/full (accessed March 26, 2022).

Persad, G., E. J. Emanuel, S. Sangenito, A. Glickman, S. Phillips, and E. A. Largent. 2021. Public perspectives on COVID-19 vaccine prioritization. *JAMA Network Open* 4(4):e217943.

Raschke, R. A., S. Agarwal, P. Rangan, C. W. Heise, and S. C. Curry. 2021. Discriminant accuracy of the SOFA score for determining the probable mortality of patients with COVID-19 pneumonia requiring mechanical ventilation. *JAMA* 325(14):1469-1470.

Rushton C. H., T. A. Thomas, I. M. Antonsdottir, K. E. Nelson, D. Boyce, A. Vioral, D. Swavely, C. D. Ley, and G. C. Hanson. 2021. Moral injury and moral resilience in health care workers during COVID-19 pandemic. *Journal of Palliative Medicine.* http://doi.org/10.1089/jpm.2021.0076 (accessed March 26, 2022).

Schorsch, K. 2020. During the pandemic, Chicago hospitals are on their own to transfer patients. *National Public Radio.* https://www.npr.org/local/309/2020/06/29/884635547/during-the-pandemic-chicago-hospitals-are-on-their-own-to-transfer-patients (accessed March 26, 2022).

Sederstrom, N. O., J. Wiggleton-Little. 2021. Acknowledging the Burdens of 'Blackness'. HEC forum: An interdisciplinary journal on hospitals' ethical and legal issues, 33(1-2), 19–33. https://doi.org/10.1007/s10730-021-09444-w.

Tolchin, B., S. C. Hull, and K. Kraschel. 2021. Triage and justice in an unjust pandemic: Ethical allocation of scarce medical resources in the setting of racial and socioeconomic disparities. *Journal of Medical Ethics* 47:200-202.

Wan, W. 2021. Burned out by the pandemic, 3 in 10 health-care workers consider leaving the profession. *Washington Post.* April 22. https://www.washingtonpost.com/health/2021/04/22/health-workers-covid-quit (accessed January 26, 2022).

REFERENCES

WHO (World Health Organization). n.d. *Health workforce.* https://www.who.int/health-topics/health-workforce#tab=tab_1 (accessed December 20, 2021).

Wilder-Smith, A., and S. Osman. 2020. Public health emergencies of international concern: A historic overview. *Journal of Travel Medicine* 27(8). https://doi.org/10.1093/jtm/taaa227 (accessed March 26, 2022).

World Bank Group. 2017. *From panic and neglect to investing in health security: Financing pandemic preparedness at a national level (English).* Washington, DC: World Bank Group.

Wortham, J. M., J. T. Lee, S. Althomsons, J. Latash, A. Davidson, K. Guerra, K. Murray, E. McGibbon, C. Pichardo, B. Toro, L. Li, M. Paladini, M. L. Eddy, K. H. Reilly, L. McHugh, D. Thomas, S. Tsai, M. Ojo, S. Rolland, M. Bhat, K. Hutchinson, J. Sabel, S. Eckel, J. Collins, C. Donovan, A. Cope, B. Kawasaki, S. McLafferty, N. Alden, R. Herlihy, B. Barbeau, A. C. Dunn, C. Clark, P. Pontones, M. L. McLafferty, D. E. Sidelinger, A. Krueger, L. Kollmann, L. Larson, S. Holzbauer, R. Lynfield, R. Westergaard, R. Crawford, L. Zhao, J. M. Bressler, J. S. Read, J. Dunn, A. Lewis, G. Richardson, J. Hand, T. Sokol, S. H. Adkins, B. Leitgeb, T. Pindyck, T. Eure, K. Wong, D. Datta, G. D. Appiah, J. Brown, R. Traxler, E. H. Koumans, and S. Reagan-Steiner. 2020. Characteristics of persons who died with COVID-19, United States, February 12–May 18, 2020. *Morbidity and Mortality Weekly Report* 69(28):923-929.

Wrigley-Field, E., M. V. Kiang, A. R. Riley, M. Barbieri, Y.-H. Chen, K. A. Duchowny, E. C. Matthay, D. V. Riper, K. Jegathesan, K. Bibbins-Domingo, and J. P. Leider. 2021. Geographically targeted COVID-19 vaccination is more equitable and averts more deaths than age-based thresholds alone. *Science Advances* 7(40):eabj2099.

Appendix A

Workshop Agendas

Webinar 1:
*Evolving Crisis Standards of Care:
Reflections, Inflections and the Future*

September 27, 2021
12–2 pm ET

12:00pm	**Opening Remarks** **Eric Toner,** Senior Scholar, Johns Hopkins University
12:10pm	**Sponsor's Charge** **Dan Hanfling,** Vice President, Technical Staff, In-Q-Tel
12:15pm	**CSC—The First Ten Years** **Dan Hanfling,** Vice President, Technical Staff, In-Q-Tel
12:40pm	**Keynote Commentary—CSC & COVID-19** **Craig Vanderwagen,** Rear Admiral USPHS—retired, founding Assistant Secretary for Preparedness and Response (ASPR) at the U.S. Department of Health and Human Services, and Founder and General Manager of East West Protection, LLC
12:55pm	**BREAK**

1:00pm	**Panel Discussion and Q&A** **Monica Peek,** Professor of Medicine, University of Chicago Medicine **Jennifer Piatt,** Deputy Director with the Network for Public Health Law's Western Region Office **Mike Wargo,** VP for Preparedness & Emergency Operations, HCA Healthcare's enterprise **Anuj Mehta,** Assistant Professor, University of Colorado **Dan Hanfling,** Vice President, Technical Staff, In-Q-Tel
1:55pm	**Closing Statement** Eric Toner, Senior Scholar, Johns Hopkins University

Webinar 2:
Evolving CSC: Staffing Considerations, Workforce Impacts, and Future Trends

October 11, 2021
12:00–2:20pm ET

12:00pm	**Opening Remarks** Eric Toner, Senior Scholar, Senior Scientist, Center for Health Security, Johns Hopkins University
12:05pm	**Stakeholders & Considerations** Asha Devereaux, M.D., M.P.H., Pulmonary Physician, ACCP Task Force for Mass Critical Care, CAL-MAT, Sr. Medical Officer, Sharp Coronado Hospital
12:15pm	**Workforce Impacts of COVID-19: A Presentation Followed by a Panel Discussion** Asha Devereaux (**Moderator**), Pulmonary Physician, ACCP Task Force for Mass Critical Care, CAL-MAT, Sr. Medical Officer, Sharp Coronado Hospital *Presentation* **Jeanette Ives Erickson,** Chief Nurse Emerita, Massachusetts General Hospital, Instructor at Harvard Medical School, and Professor at MGH Institute of Health Professions

Panel Discussion & Q&A
- **Andrew Garrett,** Associate Professor, George Washington University; Senior Advisor, Office of Emergency Management and Medical Operation, ASPR/HHS
- **Gamunu Wijetunge,** Emergency Medical Services Specialist, Office of EMS, NHTSA
- **Cynda Hylton Rushton,** Anne and George L. Bunting Professor of Clinical Ethics, Berman Institute of Bioethics, School of Nursing at Johns Hopkins University
- **Jeanette Ives Erickson,** Chief Nurse Emerita, Massachusetts General Hospital, Instructor at Harvard Medical School, and Professor at MGH Institute of Health Professions

1:00pm   BREAK

1:10pm   Promising Strategies & Future Directions
Asha Devereaux, (Moderator) Pulmonary Physician, ACCP Task Force for Mass Critical Care, CAL-MAT, Sr. Medical Officer, Sharp Coronado Hospital

Panel Discussion & Q&A
- **Lisa Rowen,** Chief Nurse Executive, University of Maryland Medical System
- **Ryan Maves,** Professor, Infectious Diseases, Wake Forest School of Medicine,
- **Howard Backer,** Medical Director, California Medical Assistance Teams, California EMSA
- **Alistair Erskine,** Chief Digital Health Officer, Mass General Brigham
- **Alexander Niven,** Associate Professor, Pulmonary and Critical Care Medicine, the Mayo Clinic, Rochester, MN

2:05pm   Planning Committee Reflections
- **Eric Toner, (Moderator)** Senior Scholar, Senior Scientist, Center for Health Security, Johns Hopkins University
- **Asha Devereaux,** Pulmonary Physician, ACCP Task Force for Mass Critical Care, CAL-MAT, Sr. Medical Officer, Sharp Coronado Hospital
- **Tener Goodwin Veenema, Ph.D., M.P.H., M.S., R.N., FAAN,** Contributing Scholar and Professor of Nursing, Johns Hopkins Center for Health Security, Johns Hopkins Bloomberg School of Public Health

2:15pm   Closing Statement
Eric Toner, (**Moderator**) Senior Scholar, Senior Scientist, Center for Health Security, Johns Hopkins University

Webinar 3:
Evolving CSC: "From Plans to Reality"

October 25, 2021
12:00–2:15pm ET

12:00pm   Opening Remarks
Eric Toner, Senior Scholar, Senior Scientist, Center for Health Security, Johns Hopkins University

12:05pm   Setting the Stage
- **John Hick, (Moderator)** Professor of Emergency Medicine, University of Minnesota
- **Anuj Mehta**, Assistant Professor of Medicine, Denver Health and Hospital Authority, University of Colorado, National Jewish Health

12:15pm   Implementation Cases Stories
- **John Hick, (Moderator)** Professor of Emergency Medicine, University of Minnesota
- **Gina Febbraro**, Planning and Improvement Consultant and Coach Prevention Services Division, Colorado Department of Public Health & Environment
- **Chris Emory**, Chief for the Bureau of Health Emergency Management (BHEM), Epidemiology and Response Division, New Mexico Department of Health (NMDOH)
- **Elizabeth Chuang**, Albert Einstein College of Medicine Montefiore Medical Center

1:00pm   **BREAK**

1:10pm   Exploring Challenges—Flash Discussion Rounds
John Hick, (Moderator) Professor of Emergency Medicine, University of Minnesota

Panel 1: Workforce Preparation Challenges (15 min)
- **Emily Kidd**, Medical Director for the Acadian Ambulance in San Antonio, TX

- Erin Talati Paquett, Assistant Professor, Pediatrics (critical care), and School of Law, Northwestern University

Panel 2: Decision Making Challenges (15 min)
- Brian Garibaldi, Associate Professor of Medicine, Johns Hopkins Biocontainment Unit
- Vikramjit Mukherjee, Medical Director, Special Pathogens Program, Bellevue Hospital Center, Director, Medical Intensive Care Unit (MICU), Bellevue Hospital Center

Panel 3: Public and Stakeholder Perceptions (20 min)
- Elizabeth Lee Daugherty, Chief Wellness Officer, Associate Professor of Medicine, Johns Hopkins Medicine
- Will Stone, Science reporter, NPR
- Julie Reiskin, Executive Director of the Colorado Cross-Disability Coalition (CCDC)

2:00pm   Planning Committee Reflections
John Hick, (**Moderator**) Professor of Emergency Medicine, University of Minnesota
- Eric Toner, Senior Scholar, Senior Scientist, Center for Health Security, Johns Hopkins University
- Anuj Mehta, Assistant Professor of Medicine, Denver Health and Hospital Authority, University of Colorado, National Jewish Health
- Erin Serino, Deputy Chief of Staff, Boston Emergency Medical Services
- Shandiin Wood, Health Systems Epidemiologist & Tribal Liaison, New Mexico Department of Health
- Megan Jehn, Ph.D., Associate Professor, Arizona State University

2:10pm   Closing Statement
Eric Toner, M.D., Senior Scholar, Senior Scientist, Center for Health Security, Johns Hopkins University

Webinar 4:
Evolving CSC: "Legal, Ethical and Equity Considerations"

November 8, 2022
12:00–2:15pm ET

12:00pm　Opening Remarks
Eric Toner, Senior Scholar, Senior Scientist, Center for Health Security, Johns Hopkins University

12:05pm　Liability Protections: Issues around Making Triage Decisions

Main Presentation
- **Monica Peek, (Moderator)** Professor of Medicine, University of Chicago
- **James Hodge, (Main Presenter)** Peter Kiewit Foundation Professor of Law, Sandra Day O'Connor College of Law; and Director, Center for Public Health Law and Policy, Arizona State University [7–8 min]

Panel Discussants
- **Robert Onders,** Alaska Native Medical Center Administrator, Alaska Native Tribal Health Consortium
- **Valerie Gutmann Koch,** co-director of the Health Law & Policy Institute, Houston Law Center; and Director of Law & Ethics at the University of Chicago MacLean Center for Clinical Medical Ethics
- **Doug White,** Vice Chair and Professor of Critical Care Medicine, UPMC Endowed Chair for Ethics in Critical Care Medicine, Director, Program on Ethics and Decision Making in Critical Illness, University of Pittsburgh School of Medicine
- **James Hodge,** Peter Kiewit Foundation Professor of Law, Sandra Day O'Connor College of Law; and Director, Center for Public Health Law and Policy, Arizona State University

12:50pm　BREAK [10 min]

APPENDIX A   83

1:00pm   Equity & the Allocations of Scarce Resources

            Main Presentation
            - **Monica Peek, (Moderator)** Professor of Medicine, University of Chicago
            - **Govind Persad,** Assistant Professor, Sturm College of Law

            Panel Discussants
            - **Nneka Sederstrom,** Chief Health Equity Officer, Hennepin Healthcare
            - **Virginia A. Brown,** Assistant Professor, Department of Population Health, Dell Medical School, The University of Texas at Austin
            - **Thomas Sequist,** Chief Patient Experience and Equity Officer at Mass General Brigham
            - **Govind Persad,** Assistant Professor, Sturm College of Law

1:55pm   Reflections

            Aims: *Highlight key takeaways and reflection from session and connect to future/final session*
            - **Monica Peek, (Moderator)** Professor of Medicine, University of Chicago
            - **Suzet McKinney,** Principle & Director, Life Sciences
            - **Jennifer Piatt,** Deputy Director, Network for Public Health Law's Western Region Office
            - **Cynda Rushton,** Professor and Chair, Johns Hopkins School of Nursing

2:12pm   Closing Statement
            Eric Toner, Senior Scholar, Senior Scientist, Center for Health Security, Johns Hopkins University

Webinar 5:

Evolving CSC: Looking Forward

November 22, 2021
12:00–2:15pm ET

12:00pm   Opening Remarks
            Eric Toner, Senior Scholar, Senior Scientist, Center for Health Security, Johns Hopkins University

12:05pm   Keynote Address
- **David Christian Hassell,** Senior Science Advisor, Deputy Assistant Secretary for Preparedness and Response, Office of the Assistant Secretary for Preparedness and Response, US/HHS
- **Richard Hunt,** Senior Medical Advisor, National Health Care Preparedness Programs, Office of the Assistant Secretary for Preparedness and Response, US/HHS

12:25pm   Staffing Considerations: Reflection on Challenges & Opportunities
- **Asha Devereaux,** Pulmonary Physician, ACCP Task Force for Mass Critical Care, CAL-MAT, Sr. Medical Officer, Sharp Coronado Hospital
- **Tener Goodwin Veenema,** Contributing Scholar and Professor of Nursing Johns Hopkins Center for Health Security Johns Hopkins Bloomberg School of Public Health
- **Mike Wargo,** VP & Chief, Enterprise Preparedness & Emergency Operations, HCA Healthcare
- **Gregg Meyers,** President of the Community Division & Executive Vice President of Value Based Care, Mass General Brigham

12:50pm   BREAK [10 min]

1:00pm   Planning and Implementation: Reflection on Challenges & Opportunities
- **Anuj Mehta,** Assistant Professor of Medicine, Denver Health and Hospital Authority, University of Colorado, National Jewish Health
- **Erin Serino,** Deputy Chief of Staff, Boston Emergency Medical Services
- **Shandiin Wood,** Health Systems Epidemiologist & Tribal Liaison, New Mexico Department of Health

1:25pm   Legal, Ethical, and Equity: Reflection on Challenges & Opportunities
- **Monica Peek,** Professor of Medicine, University of Chicago
- **Matt Wynia,** Director, Center for Bioethics and Humanities, University of Colorado

APPENDIX A 85

- **Jennifer Piatt,** Deputy Director, Network for Public Health Law's Western Region Office

1:50pm Looking to Future
- **Eric Toner,** Senior Scholar, Senior Scientist, Center for Health Security, Johns Hopkins University
- **Suzet McKinney,** Principle & Director, Life Sciences
- **Dan Hanfling,** Vice President, Technical Staff, In-Q-Tel
- **Matt Wynia,** Director, Center for Bioethics and Humanities, University of Colorado

2:10pm Closing Statement
Eric Toner, Senior Scholar, Senior Scientist, Center for Health Security, Johns Hopkins University

Appendix B

Speaker Biosketches

Howard Backer, M.D., M.P.H., was appointed CAL-MAT Medical Director in July 2011. Dr. Howard Backer received a bachelor of science degree from the University of Michigan, a master of public health degree from the University of California, Berkeley, and a doctor of medicine from the University of California, San Francisco. Dr. Backer practiced emergency medicine in private practice for 25 years before entering public service. The doctor served in a number of positions from 2000 to 2008 at the state Department of Health Services, including chief of immunization. He became associate secretary for emergency preparedness at the Health and Human Services Agency in 2008 before being tapped as the interim director at the Department of Public Health early in 2011. By statute, the EMSA director must be a physician with experience in emergency training. Reflecting a lifelong interest in wilderness and travel medicine, Dr. Backer is a founding member of the Wilderness Medical Society and a fellow of the Academy of Wilderness Medicine. He also is medical consultant for an international adventure travel company and is an expert in field water disinfection and infectious diseases of travelers. He still works clinical hours in Urgent Care at the University of California, Berkeley Student Health Center.

Virginia A. Brown, Ph.D., M.A., currently serves as an Assistant Professor in the Division of Community Engagement and Health Equity in the Department of Population Health of the University of Texas at Austin. She holds a courtesy appointment in the Department of Psychiatry at Dell Medical, and she serves as the Associate Director of Liberal Arts Honors (LAH) in the College of Liberal Arts. Her research work focuses on protecting the autonomy of persons living with serious mental illness using psychiatric advance directives (PADs), which are a communication tool that promotes patient autonomy and provides capacitated adults, who live with serious mental illnesses, the ability to record their preferences for care as well as the ability to designate a proxy decision maker before a health care crisis occurs. Currently she is working to implement PADs as within the SAMHSAs Assisted Outpatient Treatment project awarded to Integral Care, Austin's local mental health authority. In her work, Dr. Brown addresses inequity in research by applying a community based participatory research (CBPR) framework to her work, which uses a range of methodological approaches to center the priorities, the experiences, the strengths, and the knowledge communities have in identifying and solving health and health care related problems. In her current work, funded by the Patient Centered Outcomes Institute's (PCORI) Eugene Washington PCORI Engagement Award, she and her team along with a group of community partners collaborated to develop Citizen Scientist Training to serve as the foundation for establishing community and academic research partnerships for research focused on mental health. By shifting to collaboration to co-create research practice we can establish an ethical social justice framework for addressing inequality in health and health care.

Elizabeth Chuang, M.D., joined the faculty of the Department of Family and Social Medicine at Albert Einstein College of Medicine Montefiore Medical Center in 2013 after completing a fellowship in Hospice and Palliative Medicine at Montefiore. She practices hospice and palliative medicine on the inpatient consult service and palliative care inpatient unit at Montefiore Medical Center. In 2018, she joined the Montefiore-Einstein Center for Bioethics as a bioethics consultant. Dr. Chuang's research interests include clinician implicit bias, reducing racial and ethnic disparities at the end of life and clinical communication and decision-making. Dr. Chuang also enjoys teaching medical students, residents, fellows and faculty principles of bioethics, research ethics and approaches to emotionally difficult communication tasks.

Elizabeth Lee Daugherty Biddison, M.D., M.P.H., is Associate Professor of Medicine in the Johns Hopkins Division of Pulmonary and Critical Care Medicine and Chief Wellness Officer for Johns Hopkins Medicine. She is Associate Faculty in the Johns Hopkins Armstrong Institute for Patient Safety and Quality and a Contributing Scholar in the Johns Hopkins Center for Health Security. Dr. Daugherty Biddison's research interests include hospital operations, patient safety, critical care disaster response, and physician well-being. In addition to her research responsibilities, Dr. Daugherty Biddison also serves as Vice Chair for Clinical Affairs for Department of Medicine in the Johns Hopkins School of Medicine. She chairs the Department's Clinical Directors Council and co-chairs the Clinical Affairs Planning and Strategy team. She also serves as a member of the Johns Hopkins Hospital's Credentials Committee. Immediately prior to becoming Chief Wellness Officer, she served on the Dean's Task Force on Joy in Medicine. As part of that work, she co-chaired the Working Group on Culture and Work-life Balance and served as lead author of the summary report of the Task Force. She currently represents Johns Hopkins on the National Academy of Medicine Action Collaborative on Clinician Well-Being and Resilience. Dr. Daugherty Biddison completed her undergraduate studies in journalism at Washington and Lee University, magna cum laude, and received her medical degree from Georgetown University School of Medicine, cum laude. She is a member of the Phi Beta Kappa and Alpha Omega Alpha Honor Societies. She completed her internal medicine residency at the University of Pennsylvania and her Pulmonary and Critical Care Medicine fellowship at Johns Hopkins, where she also earned her Master of Public Health degree.

Chris Emory, M.S., is an Ohio native who relocated to Santa Fe, New Mexico from Western North Carolina after a 7-year residence there. Mr. Emory is the Bureau Chief for the Bureau of Health Emergency Management (BHEM), with the Epidemiology and Response Division, at the New Mexico Department of Health (NMDOH). For nearly 6 years, Chris has helped move NMDOH and the state forward in emergency planning and preparedness. The Bureau is responsible for all of New Mexico's public health and hospital preparedness and response activities, as well as the provision of strategic direction, support, and coordination for these activities across the state. Prior to the position in New Mexico, Chris was actively involved in public health preparedness in North Carolina while working as an independent contractor with local jurisdictions in Asheville and surrounding areas. He lead preparedness efforts focusing on at-risk populations by building lasting partnerships and facilitating a team planning environment, incorporating partners from government, community-based, faith-based, industry, and civic organizations. This at-risk populations' work that Chris developed was reviewed by the UNC Institute for Public Health and adopted as a toolkit for other jurisdictions to follow. Chris received his B.S. in applied science from Youngstown State University, his M.S. in public health from Touro University, and an all but dissertation Ph.D. in epidemiology from Walden University.

Jeanette Ives Erickson, R.N., D.N.P., NEA-BC, FAAN, is chief nurse emerita at Massachusetts General Hospital, Instructor at Harvard Medical School, and Professor at the MGH Institute of Health Professions. She also serves as the chair, Chief Nurse Council, Mass General Brigham. Dr. Ives Erickson earned her diploma in nursing from Mercy Hospital School of Nursing, her B.S.N. from Westbrook College, her M.S. from Boston University, and her doctorate of executive nursing practice from the MGH Institute of Health Professions. She is a Fellow in the American Academy of Nursing and a past Robert Wood Johnson Executive Nurse Fellow where her research was the role of the Chief Nurse in integrated health care systems. While fostering nursing research within an interdisciplinary, professional practice model, Dr. Ives Erickson has developed new measures to evaluate innovations that influence professional nursing practice. Along with colleagues she has developed The Professional Practice Environment scale that is used to evaluate nurses' and other clinicians' perceptions and satisfaction with the professional practice environment in which they work. This instrument is being used by more than 100 healthcare institutions, in 15 countries, and has been translated into multiple languages including Chinese, Finnish, Turkish and Spanish. She has published three books to advance nursing practice, research and the importance of a narrative culture. In addition, as part of the MGH celebration of its 200th anniversary, she and colleagues published the History of MGH Nursing. All four books have won awards. Dr. Ives Erickson is a member of the Commission on Magnet Recognition. She is the inaugural incumbent of the Paul M Erickson Endowed Chair in Nursing at the Massachusetts General Hospital. Dr. Ives Erickson serves as vice chair of the Board of Trustees for the MGH Institute of Health Professions and is co-chair of the Lunder-Dineen Health Education Alliance of Maine. Since 2008, she has been the lead nurse consultant for the strategic collaboration in the creation of Jiahui International Hospital (JIH) in China's Shanghai Province.

Alistair Erskine, M.D., is the Chief Digital Health Officer at Mass General Brigham, which includes teaching hospitals for Harvard Medical School. He is responsible for sequencing innovative technologies, harmonizing data across the clinical care, research and health plan enterprise, and activating patients in a manner congruent with emerging patient consumerism. Dr. Erskine heads Mass General Brigham Digital Health division, including the Electronic Health Record (eCare), Health Information Management/Interoperability, Virtual Care with more than 550 staff. He also leads Mass General Brigham's digital health strategy including patient-facing application, patient relationship management, telehealth services, and secondary use of data and appropriate application of artificial intelligence. He has a teaching appointment at Harvard Medical School to incorporate clinical informatics into the medical student curriculum. Prior to Mass General Brigham, Dr. Erskine was Geisinger Health System's Chief Informatics Officer where he oversaw Geisinger's Unified Data Architecture, a hedged data management environment powered by Hadoop/Big Data and traditional relational database systems to ensure that data collected as a by-product of clinical and research investigation are accessible for new discovery and appropriate secondary use. In previous roles, he was appointed Associate Dean of Medical Informatics at Virginia Commonwealth University and was a member of the Board for the 650-physician Medical College of Physician practice plan. He was appointed to the Virginia Governor's Health Information Technology Commission by Executive Order and was a voting member of the Health Information Technology Standards Committee. Dr. Erskine spent 2 years in Doha, Qatar in the Middle East as Chief of Health Informatics at Sidra Medical and Research Center and implemented a model commercial EHR from the ground up, without legacy systems or technologies. He presents and publishes on the topic of clinical transformation in peer-reviewed literature and serves on Boards of several companies. Dr. Erskine trained at Brown University and Virginia Commonwealth University Health System and is triple Board-Certified in Internal Medicine, Clinical Informatics and Pediatrics. He completed a 2-year degree program at MIT Sloan School of Management, with a specialization in Business Analytics and Artificial Intelligence. He has been practicing hospital medicine for 15 years.

Gina Febbraro, M.P.H., serves as the Planning and Improvement Consultant for the Prevention Services Division at the Colorado Department of Public Health and Environment (CDPHE) in addition to leading her own consulting business, Summit Cove Consultants LLC. For the past 8 years, Gina has advised and supported senior leadership and prevention programs in assessment, strategic planning, change management, performance management and quality improvement. Prior to this role, Gina served as the Maternal and Child Health Program (MCH) Manager for 5 years where she managed the day-to-day operations of the MCH Program including the administration of funds to local public health agencies throughout the state. Gina also served as the director of the Tony Grampsas Youth Services Program, a state-legislated grant program that funds more than 100 community-based, youth-serving organizations throughout Colorado. Before CDPHE, Gina developed community partnerships and award-winning sexuality education programs for Girls Inc. of Metro Denver. Gina earned her Master's of Public Health in health behavior and health education from the University of North Carolina's Gillings School of Public Health and her Bachelor's degree in social psychology from the Pennsylvania State University.

Brian Garibaldi, M.D., is an associate professor in the Division of Pulmonary and Critical Care Medicine, where he attends in the Medical Intensive Care Unit (MICU) and the Interstitial Lung Disease clinic. He is medical director of the Johns Hopkins Biocontainment Unit (BCU), a federally-funded special pathogens treatment center. He is also the associate program director of the Osler Medical Residency Program, where he leads curriculum development and implementation. Dr. Garibaldi was instrumental in creating the Johns Hopkins BCU. He helped to design the physical structure of the unit, created the physician-staffing model and constructed the clinical care guidelines and protocols. He also led the design of the BCU simulation and training program for the care of patients with highly infectious diseases. He has an in-depth knowledge of the challenges of the biocontainment environment and understands the specific threats to both health care worker and patient safety in the setting of highly infectious diseases. In addition to caring for patients with COVID-19, he is the director of the newly established COVID-19 Precision Medicine Center of Excellence, which houses the JH-CROWN clinical registry. He is a fellow of the New York Academy of Medicine, the Royal College of Physicians of Edinburgh and the American College of Physicians. He is also a member of the Miller-Coulson Academy of Clinical Excellence. Dr. Garibaldi grew up in New York City and graduated summa cum laude from Harvard College with a degree in biological anthropology. Before earning his medical degree from the Johns Hopkins University School of Medicine, he spent a year studying flamenco and classical guitar in Spain as part of the John Finley Fellowship from Harvard College.

Andrew Garrett, M.D., M.P.H., is the academic section chief for Emergency Health Operations and is an associate professor at George Washington University's School for Medicine and Health Sciences. His medical specialties are pediatrics, as well as EMS and disaster medicine. He is also board certified in these areas. Dr. Garrett has more than 15 years of leadership experience with the federal disaster response community and has spent much of his career with the Department of Health and Human Services (HHS) as the chief medical officer and then director of the National Disaster Medical System (NDMS), overseeing a system of nearly 7,000 federal employees and more than 80 medical, veterinary, and mass fatality disaster response teams. He also spent 2 years at the White House, most recently as the director for Biodefense and Medical Preparedness on the National Security Council. He also serves as senior adviser to the Office of Emergency Management and Medical Operations (ASPR/HHS). He has deployed both domestically and internationally to over 20 major disasters and public health emergencies, as both a clinical provider and as the chief medical officer to the federal government's Health and Public Health Incident command structure.

Valerie Gutmann Koch, J.D., is co-director of the Health Law & Policy Institute. She also serves as the Director of Law & Ethics at the University of Chicago MacLean Center for Clinical Medical Ethics. Previously, she was the Jaharis Faculty Fellow at DePaul University College of Law and a Visiting Assistant Professor at IIT Chicago-Kent College of Law. Professor Koch was the Special Advisor and Senior Attorney to the New York State Task Force on Life and the Law, the state's bioethics commission, where she crafted policy and guidance related to pandemic preparedness and crisis standards of care, human subjects research, and surrogate decision-making. Following law school, she practiced in the intellectual property litigation practice at Kirkland & Ellis LLP. As a scholar of bioethics, public policy, and health law, Professor Koch concentrates on how medical and technological advances have informed and sometimes transformed various areas of law, identifying ways in which law and policy is—or is not—equipped to address changes in technology and practice. She earned her J.D. degree from Harvard Law School, where she was the co-editor of the recent developments section of the *Journal of Law, Medicine & Ethics*. She graduated magna cum laude from Princeton University, with an A.B. from the Princeton School of Public and International Affairs, with a focus in bioethics. Professor Koch is committed to public service, including serving as the Chair of the ABA's Special Committee on Bioethics and the Law and Co-Chair of the Law Affinity Group for the American Society for Bioethics and the Humanities.

David Christian "Chris" Hassell, Ph.D., is the Senior Science Advisor and Deputy Assistant Secretary within the Office of the Assistant Secretary for Preparedness and Response in the U.S. Department of Health and Human Services. He recently served as the Deputy Assistant Secretary of Defense for Chemical and Biological Defense, where he led research, development, testing, and acquisition of technical solutions to counter chemical and biological threats. Prior to joining the Department of Defense, Dr. Hassell was an Assistant Director of the Federal Bureau of Investigation (FBI), where he served as Director of the FBI Laboratory and Executive Champion for LGBT concerns. He had previously held research and leadership positions at Los Alamos National Laboratory and DuPont. Dr. Hassell is an analytical chemist with specialization in sensors, diagnostics and bioprocessing, and is a Fellow of the Society for Applied Spectroscopy. He is a recipient of the Defense Medal for Exceptional Civilian Service (US) and the Médaille de la Défense Nationale (France).

Richard C. Hunt, M.D., FACEP, is ASPR's Senior Medical Advisor for National Healthcare Preparedness Programs. From 2013 to 2015, he served The White House as Director for Medical Preparedness Policy, National Security Staff. During this time, he played a critical role in the response to the Ebola crisis and led the "Stop the Bleed" initiative. Prior to his positions in Washington, DC, Dr. Hunt was Distinguished Consultant and Director of the Division of Injury Response at CDC's National Center for Injury Prevention and Control. Prior to federal service, he served as professor and chair of the Department of Emergency Medicine at SUNY Upstate Medical University in Syracuse, New York. He is a past president of the National Association of EMS Physicians. Dr. Hunt is board certified in emergency medicine and is an adjunct professor of emergency medicine at Emory University School of Medicine.

Emily Kidd, M.D., attended Texas A&M University (B.S.), The University of Texas Health Science Center at Houston (M.D.), The Brody School of Medicine at East Carolina University (residency), and The University of Texas Health Science Center in Houston/Houston Fire Department (fellowship). She is double-board certified in both Emergency Medicine and EMS, and has been practicing emergency medicine for more than 21 years and pre-hospital (EMS) medicine for more than 16 years. She served as an Assistant Medical Director for the Houston Fire Department and as an Assistant Medical Director and Interim Medical Director for the San Antonio Fire Department. Since 2016, she has served as the Texas Medical Director for Acadian Ambulance Service. Dr. Kidd is also very actively involved in disaster and emergency management at the local, regional, state, and national levels. She was involved in field response and medical direction during Hurricanes Katrina, Rita, Gustav, Ike, and Harvey as well as the H1N1 pandemic, Ebola crisis, West, Texas explosion, and of course the COVID pandemic and recent Texas ice storm from Winter Storm Uri. Dr. Kidd held a position on FEMA's National Advisory Council for 6 years, has sat on the Governor's EMS and Trauma Advisory Council Disaster Committee for more than 14 years, and serves as the State Medical Director for the Texas Emergency Medical Task Force. She was recently elected to the position of President-Elect for the Texas Chapter of the National Association of EMS Physicians

Ryan C. Maves M.D., FCCM, FCCP, FIDSA, is professor of medicine and anesthesiology at the Wake Forest School of Medicine in Winston-Salem, North Carolina, where he serves as a faculty intensivist and infectious diseases specialist at Wake Forest Baptist Medical Center. A graduate of the University of Washington School of Medicine, he completed his internal medicine residency and fellowships in infectious diseases and critical care medicine at the Naval Medical Center in San Diego, California. Following fellowship, he served at the Naval Medical Research Unit No. 6 in Lima, Peru, leading studies in antimicrobial drug resistance and vaccine development. He returned to NMCSD in 2010, serving as ID division head. In 2012, Dr. Maves deployed to the NATO Role 3 Multinational Medical

Unit at Kandahar Airfield, Afghanistan, as Director of Medical Services. After returning from deployment, he later served as vice chair of medicine and ID fellowship program director. He was the U.S. Department of Defense coordinating principal investigator (PI) for the NIAID-sponsored Adaptive COVID-19 Treatment Trial (ACTT) and the San Diego site PI for the AstraZeneca/Oxford phase 3 ChAdOx1 SARS-CoV-2 vaccine trial. He retired from the United States Navy with the rank of Captain in 2021 after 22 years of active-duty service and joined the faculty at Wake Forest. Dr. Maves is board-certified in internal medicine, infectious diseases, and critical care medicine. He is the vice chair of the Fundamental Disaster Management committee in the Society of Critical Care Medicine and is the chair of the American College of Chest Physician's COVID-19 Task Force.

Gregg S. Meyer, M.D., MSc, is the President of the Community Division & Executive Vice President of Value Based Care for the Mass General Brigham health care system. He is responsible for two of Mass General Brigham's hospitals—Newton-Wellesley Hospital and North Shore Medical Center—where he previously served as interim President, as well as Mass General Brigham Home Care and Mass General Brigham Community Physicians. Dr. Meyer is also responsible for building and leading a best-in-class Value Based Care Program by leveraging Mass General Brigham's health insurance organization—AllWays Health Partners—and the Population Health Management initiatives across Mass General Brigham's academic medical centers, community hospitals, primary care physicians and ambulatory care and urgent care sites. Previously, Dr. Meyer was the Chief Clinical Officer of Mass General Brigham. In this role, he was responsible for the overall direction, operations and management of system aspects of health care delivery throughout the Mass General Brigham system. Dr. Meyer is also a professor of medicine at Massachusetts General Hospital and Harvard Medical School. Before returning to Mass General Brigham, Dr. Meyer served as the Chief Clinical Officer and Executive Vice-President for Population Health at Dartmouth-Hitchcock Medical Center and the Senior Associate Dean for Clinical Affairs and Paul B. Batalden Professor and Chair at the Geisel School of Medicine. Prior to going to Dartmouth-Hitchcock, Dr. Meyer served as Senior Vice President for the Edward P. Lawrence Center for Quality and Safety at the Massachusetts General Hospital and Massachusetts General Physicians Organization (MGPO). A national leader in the area of quality and safety, Dr. Meyer led the multi-faceted efforts of the MGH/MGPO in quality and safety. He also led the care redesign efforts at Mass General, which aim to improve both the quality and efficiency of care for common clinical conditions and chaired the committee charged with defining the future of clinical information systems for Partners HealthCare (now Mass General Brigham). Dr. Meyer was previously the Director of the Center for Quality Improvement and Patient Safety at the Agency for Healthcare Research and Quality (AHRQ). Before his tenure at AHRQ, Dr. Meyer was an Associate Professor at the Uniformed Services University of the Health Sciences (USUHS) where he served as Division Director for General Medicine. While at USUHS, Dr. Meyer was an active duty Medical Corps officer and Colonel in the United States Air Force. Dr. Meyer graduated from Union College and Albany Medical College. He earned a master's degree at Oxford where he was a Rhodes Scholar and holds a master's degree from Harvard. He has served on numerous national and international committees related to health care quality and safety and has authored more than 100 articles, editorials, chapters and monographs.

Vikramjit Mukherjee, M.D., is a physician at New York University School of Medicine. Dr. Mukherjee is assistant professor in the New York University (NYU) Grossman School of Medicine and director of the Medical Intensive Care Unit (MICU) at Bellevue Hospital Center. He is trained as a pulmonary critical care physician. He is board certified in internal medicine, pulmonary disease, and critical care medicine. Dr. Mukherjee serves as a leader in the National Emerging Special Pathogens Training and Education Center (NETEC). Dr. Mukherjee completed his residency at Georgetown University School of Medicine and his fellowship in pulmonary and critical care at NYU Hospitals Center.

Alexander S. Niven, M.D., is a consultant in the Division of Pulmonary and Critical Care at Mayo Clinic and associate professor of medicine in the Mayo Clinic College of Medicine. He is currently the Education Chair for Division of Pulmonary, Critical Care, and Sleep Medicine and the Critical Care Independent Multispecialty Practice there. Dr. Niven is an at-large member of the CHEST Board of Regents and has served as both a long-standing member of its Task Force for Mass Critical Care and as chair of the CHEST Wellness Task Force over the past 20 months. His research interests include the identification of optimal education strategies to enhance individual and team performance in the intensive care unit.

Robert Onders, M.D., J.D., joined the Alaska Native Tribal Health Consortium in 2015 and currently serves as the administrator of the Alaska Native Medical Center (ANMC). Previously Dr. Onders served as medical director of community and Health Systems Improvement and President of Alaska Pacific University. Prior to joining, Dr. Onders worked as clinical director for Kodiak Area Native Association and emergency department director at West Park Hospital in Cody, Wyoming. Dr. Onders graduated from a combined 6-year bachelor of science and doctor of medicine program through Kent State University and Northeast Ohio Medical University in 1997. He completed his family medicine residency, juris doctorate, and masters of public administration with the University of Wyoming.

Govind Persad, J.D., Ph.D., is an assistant professor at the Sturm College of Law. His research interests center on the legal and ethical dimensions of health insurance, health care financing (both domestic and international), and markets in health care services, as well as professional ethics and the regulation of medical research. He has been selected as a 2018–2021 Greenwall Faculty Scholar in Bioethics for an ongoing research project on health insurance and protection against financial risk. His articles have appeared or will appear in the *George Washington Law Review*, *Emory Law Journal*, *Boston College Law Review*, and *Yale Journal of Health Policy, Law, and Ethics*, among others. He was selected as a Health Law Scholar in 2017 and as a BioIP Scholar in 2018 by the American Society of Law, Medicine and Ethics. Prior to joining the faculty at the University of Denver, Dr. Persad was an assistant professor of health policy and management at the Johns Hopkins University Bloomberg School of Public Health, where he was affiliated with the Berman Institute of Bioethics and served on the School's Institutional Review Board, and was a junior faculty fellow at Georgetown University's McDonough School of Business. He clerked for the Hon. Carlos Lucero, U.S. Court of Appeals for the Tenth Circuit, in Denver.

Julie Reiskin, LCSW, is the executive director of the Colorado Cross-Disability Coalition (CCDC). In that role, Ms. Reiskin assists other organizations with assuring real and meaningful participation by "clients" at all levels. Through CCDC and the disability community, Ms. Reiskin has gained expertise on nonprofit accountability and best practices, publically funded long-term community based services, disability rights law, public benefits, and the intersectionality of systemic and individual advocacy. Ms. Reiskin has proposed and helped to implement many solutions to create a sustainable and client friendly Medicaid program, such as the consumer direction as a delivery model, acted as a respected advocate for individuals, and has trained many others in health advocacy and health policy. Prior to becoming the executive director for CCDC in 1996, Ms. Reiskin served as the organization's policy analyst. In 2010, she was appointed by President Obama to serve on the board of directors of the Legal Services Corporation as the client representative.

Ms. Reiskin provides consulting with organizations seeking to improve, expand, or enhance their ability to effectively practice real and meaningful client/constituent engagement at all levels of the organization. She also helps organizations develop disability cultural competence. She moved to Colorado from Connecticut in 1994. In Connecticut, she was a partner in a consulting firm, specializing in diversity issues throughout Southern New England. She also had a private psychotherapy practice. Previous work includes several positions working with "hard to serve" youth and positive youth development, AIDS/HIV education, and grassroots community organizing. Ms. Reiskin has taught extensively in the areas of disability rights, disability culture, and disability policy, along with other areas related to diversity in human services. Ms. Reiskin received her master's in social work from the University of Connecticut, with a major in community organizing in 1989. She obtained a B.S. in women's studies from the University of Connecticut in 1985.

Lisa Rowen, DNSc, R.N., CENP, FAAN, is System Chief Nurse Executive for the University of Maryland Medical System. As System Chief Nurse Executive, Dr. Rowen adds a senior nursing voice at the system level for strategic planning, nursing workforce development and continuous clinical improvement initiatives. Since 2007, Dr. Rowen has served as Senior Vice President for Patient Care Services and Chief Nursing Officer (CNO) at the University of Maryland Medical Center, and in 2015 was also appointed as CNO for the University of Maryland Medical Center Midtown Campus. Dr. Rowen has oversight of more than 5,000 nurses, advanced practice nurses and other health professionals; she will continue in these roles while dedicating a portion of her time and effort to this new System role. Dr. Rowen is a member of the UMMS Board of Directors and serves as the System Chair of the UMMS Chief Nursing Officer Council, which is composed of the UMMS hospital CNOs and provides the vision for nursing across the Medical System. Under Dr. Rowen's leadership, UMMC was awarded Magnet Designation by the American Nurses Credentialing Center in 2009 and was re-credentialed in 2014. Only approximately five percent of all hospitals across the United States have achieved this prestigious designation, which recognizes hospitals that demonstrate excellence in nursing practice and adherence to national standards for nursing care. As associate professor at the University of Maryland School of Nursing, Dr. Rowen has formulated innovative relationships with the SON to advance education and training of nurses from beginning of the career through advanced nursing practices. She also holds faculty appointments at University of Virginia, the Johns Hopkins University, and Northeastern University. Dr. Rowen earned a Bachelor of Arts degree in art history and a Bachelor of Science degree in nursing at the University of Delaware, a Master of Science degree at the University of Maryland, and a Doctor of Nursing Science degree at the Johns Hopkins University. Among her professional affiliations, Dr. Rowen is a member of the American Academy of Nursing, American Organization of Nurse Executives, American Nurses Association, and the Maryland Nurses Association.

Cynda Hylton Rushton, Ph.D., R.N., FAAN, is the Anne and George L. Bunting Professor of Clinical Ethics in the Berman Institute of Bioethics and the School of Nursing at Johns Hopkins University, with a joint appointment in the School of Medicine's Department of Pediatrics. A founding member of the Berman Institute, Dr. Rushton co-chairs the Johns Hopkins Hospital's Ethics Consultation Service. An international leader in nursing ethics, in 2014 Dr. Rushton co-led the first National Nursing Ethics Summit, convened by the Johns Hopkins Berman Institute of Bioethics and School of Nursing. The Summit, supported by strategic partners from nine national nursing organizations and seven collaborating organizations, developed a Blueprint for 21st Century Nursing Ethics. The Blueprint highlights recommendations for clinical practice, education, policy and research and has been a catalyst for strategic action coinciding with the American Nurses Association 2015 designation of the "Year of Ethics." Dr. Rushton's current scholarship in clinical ethics focuses on moral distress and suffering of clinicians, the development of moral resilience, designing a culture of ethical practice, and conceptual foundations of integrity, respect, trust and compassion.

Nneka Sederstrom Ph.D., M.P.H., M.A., FCCP, FCCM, is the Chief Health Equity Officer at Hennepin Healthcare where she leads efforts in addressing health disparities, equity, and antiracism in the institution and community. She received her B.A. in philosophy from George Washington University in 2001. She began her career at the Center for Ethics at Medstar Washington Hospital Center in Washington D.C. the same year. She completed her master's degree in philosophy and public policy from Howard University in 2003 and proceeded to begin her Ph.D. studies in medical sociology and race, class, and gender inequalities at the same university. After beginning her PhD studies, she was made Director of the Center for Ethics and Director of the Spiritual Care Department. She proceeded to hold these positions until she left to join Children's Minnesota in March 2016 where she served as the Director of the Clinical Ethics Department for almost 5 years. Her Ph.D. is in sociology with concentrations in medical sociology and race, class, and gender inequality, M.P.H. in global health management, and M.A. in philosophy. She is a member of several professional societies and holds a leadership position in CHEST Medicine and the Society of Critical Care Medicine. She is a Fellow of the American College of Chest Physicians and a Fellow of the American College of Critical Care Medicine. She is widely published in Equity and Clinical Ethics and speaks regularly at national and international meetings.

Tom Sequist, M.D., M.P.H., is the Chief Patient Experience and Equity Officer at Mass General Brigham. He leads system-wide strategies for improving patient experience, quality, safety, equity, and community health. He is a practicing general internist at Brigham and Women's Hospital and is professor of medicine and professor of health care policy at Harvard Medical School. Dr. Sequist's research interests focus on quality measurement and improvement, health care equity, patient and provider education, and the innovative use of health information technology. Dr. Sequist is a member of the Taos Pueblo tribe in New Mexico and he has conducted influential health policy research to advance our understanding of health care for Native American communities. He serves as the Director of the Four Directions Summer Research Program at Brigham and Women's Hospital and the Medical Director of the Brigham and Women's Hospital Physician Outreach Program with the Indian Health Service. Dr. Sequist graduated from Cornell University with a B.S. in chemical engineering. He received his M.D. degree from Harvard Medical School and his M.P.H. degree from the Harvard School of Public Health.

Will Stone covers health and science for NPR's Science Desk. He has previously reported for public radio stations in Connecticut, Nevada, Arizona, and Washington State. He is based in Seattle, Washington, where he has tracked the pandemic since the first confirmed U.S. case of COVID-19 in January.

Erin Talati Paquette, M.D., J.D., MBe, is a pediatric critical care doctor, lawyer, and ethicist, as well as assistant professor of pediatrics at Northwestern University's Feinberg School of Medicine. She is also adjunct professor at Northwestern University's Pritzker School of Law, a Pediatric Critical Care Scientist Development Scholar, and a Public Voices Fellow with The OpEd Project. She is interested in research, advocacy, and policy development that reduces health disparities, addresses bias, racism, and other structural determinants of health and promotes social justice. Her current research involves evaluating disparities in research enrollment and participation, the use of medico-legal partnerships to address the social determinants of health, and understanding public perceptions of brain death. Additional interests include the role for conflict resolution training to improve communication in the ICU, evaluating health care access in relation to health outcomes, and studying the informed consent process for children participating in research.

Doug White, M.D., MAS, is Vice Chair, professor of critical care medicine, and the UPMC Endowed Chair for Ethics in Critical Care Medicine, as well as the Director of the Program on Ethics and Decision Making in Critical Illness at the University of Pittsburgh School of Medicine. His research program encompasses both empirical research on and normative ethical analysis of surrogate decision making for patients with life-threatening illness. He graduated summa cum laude from Dartmouth College in 1995 with a degree in English literature. He received his M.D. from UCSF in 1999 and completed a residency in Internal Medicine and a fellowship in Pulmonary and Critical Care Medicine at UCSF. While at UCSF, he also completed a Master's degree in Epidemiology and Biostatistics and a fellowship in Bioethics under Bernard Lo. He joined the faculty at UCSF in 2005 as assistant professor of medicine and core faculty of the Program on Medical Ethics. In 2009, he joined the faculty of the University of Pittsburgh in the Departments of Critical Care Medicine and Medicine as associate professor. Dr. White directs the University of Pittsburgh Program on Ethics and Decision Making in Critical Illness. He has several ongoing NIH-funded studies. He has published widely using both quantitative and qualitative methods to examine the process of surrogate decision making in intensive care units. In conducting this work, he collaborates with a multi-disciplinary group of investigators, which includes faculty with expertise in bioethics, law, philosophy, sociology, biostatistics, and health services research. His empirical research program has two central aims: (1) to identify factors that adversely affect surrogate decision making for critically ill patients and (2) to develop and test interventions to improve surrogate decision making. His normative work focuses on ethical issues that arise in intensive care units, including the allocation of scarce resources, resolving futility disputes, responding to conscience-based treatment refusals by clinicians, and developing fair processes of decision making for incapacitated patients who lack surrogate decision makers.